INJURED TO ELITE

A Guide to Empowering Yourself to
Transform Your Life After Injury

Injured to Elite Resources

Find my digital courses to see Injured to Elite in action at
www.injuredtoelite.com

Follow me on social media
Instagram: @davemmeyer
Twitter: @PLPerform
Facebook: www.facebook.com/injuredtoelite
Join Private Facebook Group: Blueprint to Performance
Send me a DM on IG to join!

Subscribe to The Injured to Elite Podcast
On All Major Podcast Apps
Including Spotify and Apple Podcasts

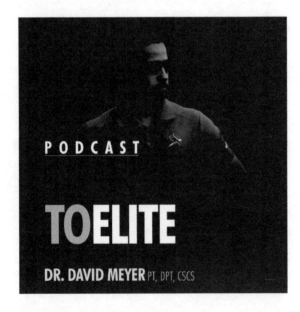

davemeyer@plperform.com

INJURED TO ELITE

A Guide to Empowering Yourself to Transform Your Life After Injury

By Dr. David Meyer PT, DPT

Foreword by Performance Coach John Denney

Published by Pipeline Performance
Plainview, New York

Library of Congress Cataloging-in-publication Data
Dr. David Meyer PT, DPT
Injured to Elite: A Guide to Empowering Yourself to Transform Your
Life After Injury
ISBN: 978-0-578-71200-0
Library of Congress Control Number: 2020914822

Author: Dr. David Meyer PT, DPT
Editor: Oleg Kagan, lifeinoleg@gmail.com
Cover Design: Rob Williams, fiverr.com/cal5086
Interior Design: Autumn Anglin, greygirlgraphics.com
Photography: Rachel Herman-Gabrielli, rhg.pics@gmail.com
Illustrations: Dr. David Meyer

Book Printing Stats: Avenir Next Condensed, Avenir Next, Georgia
Printed and Bound by KDP
Published by: Pipeline Performance
Printed in the United States of America

ISBN: 978-0-578-71200-0

Please consult with your own physician or healthcare specialist regarding the suggestions
and recommendations made in this book. The authors, editor and publisher cannot accept
responsibility for errors or exclusions or for the outcome of the application of the material
presented herein. There is no expressed or implied warranty of this book or information
imparted by it.

You understand that this book is not intended as a substitute for consultation with a
licensed healthcare practitioner, such as your physician. Before you begin any healthcare
program, or change your lifestyle in any way, you will consult your physician or another licensed healthcare practitioner to ensure that you are in good health and that the
examples contained in this book will not harm you. This book provides content related to
physical and/or mental health issues. As such, use of this book implies your acceptance of
this disclaimer.

This book is dedicated to the life of my father, Dean Meyer.

A man who went from Injured to Elite before I knew what it meant...After 2 kidney transplants, a total hip replacement, full thickness rotator cuff tear, and end-stage lung cancer (just to name a few of his illnesses), he refused to give in. I feel blessed to have been taught how to persevere through observing his experiences, and now I am honored to share what I have learned with all of you.

Share in his legacy through your own journey, going from Injured to Elite.

Use the hashtag, #injuredtoelite to join in his legacy along with the thousands of other humans that are pursuing life to its fullest after experiencing physical challenges.

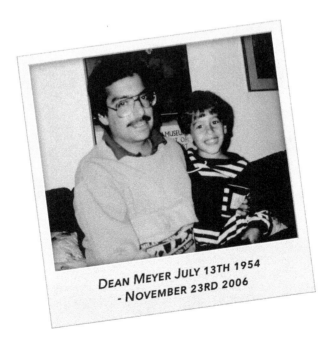

DEAN MEYER JULY 13TH 1954 - NOVEMBER 23RD 2006

#INJUREDTOELITE

CONTENTS

        Step #1: Make a conscious decision to get into the driver's seat, with the understanding that your "vehicle" is in good working order, along with trust and faith in your ability to recover.

        Step #2: Get constructive feedback from medical professionals that empowers **your** process.

        Step #3: Use biofeedback (voluntary control of autonomic bodily functions) in order to more objectively self-assess.

        Step #4: Use movement to influence your mental state.

Create and cue in your anchor switch to move forward after noting a negative thought virus.

Replace your negative thought virus with a positive thought vaccine

Part II: The Physical Body

Step #1: Follow the goldilocks "just right" principle of progression. Meet in the middle of the two extreme ideas of don't do anything in pain and "no pain no game."

Step #2: In order to manage your load and recovery, you must first know your destination and then reverse-engineer the pathway.

Step #3: Driving up the mountain after injury requires energy and momentum.

Step #4: Monitor your energy reserve in order to get you to the destination.

Steps to Diaphragmatic Breathing

Movement Self-Assessment Crash-Course

Corrective Exercises, Mobility, Stability, and Motor Control

Workload Capacity and Change of Direction

Training Fundamental Movements

Part III: Putting It All Together

FOREWORD

By John Denney, Performance Coach

I met Dr. David Meyer in 2015 and thought it was an answered prayer. He was working for the St. Louis Cardinals organization and I had been setting goals and visions to break into the baseball world as a Mental Performance Coach with my "Playing From The Heart" Program. Having had a major impact in golf, tennis, and volleyball, I knew I could make a big impact in baseball if given the opportunity. My program is designed to have a major impact in any sport that starts and stops so getting Dr. Dave into my office was going to be my golden ticket to the big leagues. I figured I would be on staff with the Cardinals shortly!

After taking him through the introductory session, showing him the best self-regulation skills I knew, scientifically-proven with the HeartMath System (high-tech biofeedback equipment that assesses heart rate variability) that I had been successfully using with many players on the PGA and LPGA tour, along with collegiate and high school teams, I was beyond excited. Well, after our session his comment was: "Yeah, I get it, but it's too spiritual for major league baseball..." Not what I was expecting, especially since the intro session does not even scratch the surface of the spiritual side of my program.

Fast forward to 2018, having long given up on my goal of breaking into baseball, I got a call from Dr. Dave asking if he should pursue a certification in HeartMath. No longer working for the Cardinals, Dr. Dave was now developing his own practice and philosophies with his company, Pipeline Performance. I noticed that he had a new open-mindedness that I had not seen when he was working for the Cardinals. I knew after that phone call that he had embraced the mental, emotional, and spiritual components and integrated them into the rehabilitation process; a steadfast belief in yourself, love for the game that you are playing, and for the people who play it with you, which are all critical components of peak performance. As you will learn in this book, *Injured to Elite*, a holistic approach to health and healing is of paramount importance.

The fact is we are not machines and cannot be repaired according to a manual. We are each a unique individual and have to be treated in a personalized way. You must believe in yourself, as you know your body and unique circumstances best. When we take care of ourselves first, mentally, physically, emotionally, and spiritually, our recovery and performance increases on every level.

In 2019, my wife and I traveled to watch our daughter play for Florida International University at the East meets West NCAA Beach Volleyball Tournament in Manhattan Beach, California. Dr. Dave and his fiancé, Olya, joined us and we spent time brainstorming and masterminding how we could incorporate more mindfulness training into the world of sports performance and rehabilitation. In many ways, this was not only an "East Meets West" volleyball tournament, but also a masterminding of eastern and western principles of establishing our health. We also met later in Marina Del Rey for a morning sunrise performance and recording of a daily Harmony Exercise guided meditation. While staying in touch over that year, and during his eventual return to New York, Dr. Dave launched the *Injured to Elite* podcast, sharing many of the ideas and concepts that you will find in this book. The podcast contains real-life stories of people going from injured to elite themselves.

"Injured To Elite" is a journey back to health, our natural condition. It is only when we are embodying perfect health that we can perform at our own personal level of elite. In this book, Dr. Dave provides us with a new and refreshing perspective on physical rehabilitation, taking us through an awakening and self-empowerment journey. He shows us why the way "they have always done it" may not be the best way forward for most people. He gives us a holistic and realistic approach to healing and restoring health.

CHAPTER 1
TIME ZERO

She hadn't been skiing for over 10 years before that day on Mount Bachelor in Bend, Oregon. It was the first day of a weekend family ski trip and after several passes down the smaller slopes she felt like she was getting the hang of it again. Finally, she worked up the courage to try one of the more advanced trails, taking the lift up a few extra stops. Halfway down, with her father carving out a path ahead, just as she started to shift her weight and actually dig the skis into the snow, carving back and forth, she began to lose control:

"...My left ski became caught and I was unable to shift my bodyweight back to the other side and so I started tumbling down the mountain. As I started rolling down, my right ski came off, but my left one remained. At one point my left knee twisted while the ski was stuck in the ground, and suddenly I heard and felt a pop which was instantly excruciating."

Dad, who was already well ahead, became concerned by his daughter's absence so he turned around, only to see his 27-year-old in the snow and unable to get up.

"Once I stopped rolling, I started yelling and crying while holding onto my knee, as a mother and son skied up to me and asked if I was okay. They asked if I was able to ski myself down, when I told them I couldn't because I was in too much pain, they went down to get help.

Ski patrol came, put me into the toboggan, and asked if I was claustrophobic since they had to zip me up into a bag to keep me safe on the sled while they skied me down the mountain to which I said yes. Since I was so high up on the mountain, they had to physically tie the toboggan onto their waist, skiing me halfway down the mountain before attaching me to a snowmobile. At that point, I couldn't tell if I was crying from physical pain or embarrassment."

Waiting down in the ski patrol medical clinic was a medical professional who happened to be a physical therapist with advanced sports medicine training. He quickly helped the women into the clinic and up on a treatment bed. After asking a series of questions, inspecting her left leg and knee, and maneuvering it into different positions and directions, he informed her that it was most likely a ligament sprain and, thankfully, it didn't seem like she fully tore any major ligaments. She sighed in relief, and they hugged.

Though this is a very typical story for many of my patients, the major difference here is that this time the patient turned out to be my significant other. At the time, we were in the middle of relocating from sunny south Florida to equally sunny southern California. At that time, my now-fiancé, Olya, was between jobs and without medical insurance. This meant that I was tasked with helping her get back on her feet. Although I have been through many more gruesome injuries with my patients and clients, this special case gave me unique insight into a person's immediate response to an injury.

A Holistic Approach

Often, the first minutes following an injury are the scariest and most confusing time for patients. In many cases, it is also a critical period to set off in the right direction on the road to recovery, especially if this isn't your first injury. Thankfully, for most people, the "worst" is usually already over.

As you'll soon see, a major theme of this book is turning a time of injury — usually associated with difficult negative feelings — into an opportunity. I will teach you how to leverage this "unfortunate event" as a momentous way to better not only your physical life, but also the other domains of your world, including your career, relationships, and overall perspective. Take it as a bit of reassurance that in your darkest hour, the only direction is towards the light; while it may seem overwhelming, you must remember that your current state of impairment is temporary, whether it be a musculoskeletal injury, a time of diagnosed systemic disease, psychological distress or mental illness, or simply a lack of physical performance.

One of the most important elements here of business is to place physical or sports performance within the context of our greater purpose; don't expect to get run-of-the-mill "bigger, faster, stronger" advice with this approach. Instead, I will give you proven methods, backed by science, on how to perform better in all areas of your life, leading to a more fulfilled mind, body, and spirit. When we take such an all-encompassing, or holistic, approach to performance, we allow for momentum in one dimension to carry over to other areas of our life. Writing about this reminds me of something my former boss, a Major League Baseball GM, once said to me: "When you look good, you feel good, when you feel good, you play good, and when you play good, you get paid good!" Clearly, the different domains of our lives do not live in isolation from one another.

It is my belief that what differentiates humans from other species is our desire to progress, which is ingrained in the human mind. When we go to sleep at night it is impossible for these ambitions not to leak into our thoughts and dreams, and when we're awake, into our conversations with friends and family. Yet, we often lack a structured approach to move forward after an injury or challenge. My approach leverages the idea that we all want to improve and teaches how to bring that about during the rehab process and beyond — it integrates rehabilitation into a unified approach to bettering oneself. That said, instead of holding your hand through this entire process like many medical professionals, coaches, and self-help gurus insist on doing, *Injured to Elite* is about the shift to becoming your own guide, not relying on a co-dependent working relationship with a so-called expert. It is about time you become the expert of your most prized material possession, your body.

Starting on the Right Path

"What just happened?" is the first question everyone asks at the very beginning of their Time Zero. If you tore a muscle, tendon, ligament, fractured a bone, suffered a head injury, are in a performance slump, or have some distracting external stresses throwing off your "game", then keep reading. If not, still keep reading! *Injured to Elite* is not meant only for those that fall into a classic injury pattern or story. It is meant for anyone dealing with adversity in their journey towards all-around peak performance. However, if you are only looking for tips about peak physical performance that will make you bigger, faster, and stronger quickly, while cutting corners and finding shortcuts, stop reading. *Injured to Elite* is not for you. Bookstores and libraries are already bursting with the stuff you want. However, if you are curious why those books haven't been transformational in your athletic career and everyday life, you'll likely find the missing pieces here.

During your darkest hour, it is the linking of all the domains in your life, and taking ownership of them, that is a necessary action to unleash your fullest potential. This book cannot force you to perform better, all it can do is lead you on the right path to make a pivotal and transformational change at a dark time in your life. Let me be your tour guide!

Acknowledging Your Present State

I have already mentioned where we are starting, which is at your darkest hour. Whether you are an athlete that is "broken", or someone in a competitive landscape that has lost your footing, or maybe you're a regular person who is tired of being blindly led around by those "in the know", we all start here. In the medical world they call the earliest time documented of triage (treatment) in an emergency setting "Time Zero". In this book, instead of referring to this time the way it might feel (for example, your darkest hour), let's call it Time Zero. Along with that adjustment, we are shifting the connotation of Time

Zero from a negative event to the beginning of your transformational journey towards peak performance and fulfillment as an athlete, high performer, and individual.

In all likelihood, you are already past your Time Zero, so it may seem like a real drag to drudge up memories of your immediate response to the injury. However, it is absolutely important to go through this in order to avoid ever returning to a Time Zero in the same way. This is not to say you will never again find yourself in a tough situation. No, part of what we are accomplishing with this transformation is making sure that next time, you will face the adversity with a different mindset; this is about turning negativity into positivity.

So unless you're so hardcore that you are lying injured on the floor and reading this book, let's take a look back to your Time Zero. I am going to help by posing some questions to bring you back to that time, much like I do when a patient comes into the clinic and gives me their history. You can write your answers down if you wish, but it's good enough that you spend a few minutes thinking and/or visualizing your responses. Here are the questions:

- ◆ What happened at your Time Zero?
- ◆ What caused your Time Zero?
- ◆ How did you feel?
- ◆ What did you say either out loud or to yourself?
- ◆ Who was there to help you?
- ◆ How did you get yourself up?
- ◆ Who did you reach out to for help?
- ◆ How did you know whom to reach out to for help?
- ◆ What was the weather that day?
- ◆ What was the first thing you were told after Time Zero?
- ◆ And maybe most importantly: What did Time Zero mean to you at the time?

The answers to these questions are going to put you in touch with the thoughts that brought you to this moment and set the stage for you to tap into the deeper aspects of your mind. Consider your responses — for most people, they're a flood of sudden challenges;

maybe the injury meant that you were going to miss time from your activity, sport, or job. Perhaps it meant that you would have to give up doing something you love. Or maybe you were terrified of the many unknowns that would follow. Maybe it meant that you were no longer whole, or that you never really felt whole...Did you think it would lead you to finding your way to a better life? Whatever your answers, it led you to this.

Note, that this may take some time and I recommend that you give yourself as much time as you need processing all of those questions. If the answers haven't connected with you on an emotional level, then keep going. I know it's tough but don't skip this area, as these are the necessary steps towards breaking through Time Zero, otherwise we might be stuck right where we started for a long time.

All too often when patients seek out my help, they know how they want to feel, but are not conscious of their current state. Of course, this means that they also don't have a clear sense of how to get to the condition they seek. For example, many patients come to me with physical musculoskeletal pain at specific regions of their body. Some have a specific goal in mind that they feel is being limited by this pain (like wanting to sleep through the night comfortably, or return to a sport), but few truly appreciate and acknowledge their total state of body, mind, and spirit. Though they may not be conscious of it, their lack of insight can serve as a real hindrance to the progress of their rehabilitation.

Which brings us back to your Time Zero. The scene is set and we are on the same page, so let's move forward.

What to Expect

Between your Time Zero and the present moment you probably went on a roller coaster that took you through many new twists and turns. During this time you either sought out others to help you, or relied on yourself to get through these unexpected circumstances. For the former, it might have been medical professionals, coaches, friends, teammates, family members, etc., while for the latter, it was likely through your own emotional coping methods and research. These days, that research was likely on the web and through social media, where you surely found a jumble of correct information and downright misinformation. A few small pieces of information alone are not enough to give you the whole picture; in the world of data, it takes many data points in order to make correlations or draw even slight conclusions. You will learn plenty more about this in chapter 3 (Conversations with Professionals) and in chapter 4 (Building Your Performance Team), where I share ways to improve your information literacy skills.

The rest of this book will take you on a journey from Injured to Elite by connecting your mind, body, and spirit from where it is now, after your Time Zero, all the way to your intended physical performance accomplishments and emotional fulfillment. Each of the following chapters will take you into an area related to your journey, from how to optimize your mindset to how you can more effectively train your body to achieve your goals.

Now that you have fully acknowledged the state that you have found yourself in after your Time Zero, it is time to dive deeper into that mind of yours by shifting your mental state to unleash the inner superhero. This will lay the foundation for the other necessary steps to take you from Injured to Elite.

#InjuredToElite

Part I: The Mind

"Baseball is 90% mental, the other half is physical."

- Yogi Berra, Hall of Fame catcher

#InjuredToElite

CHAPTER 2
TAKING OWNERSHIP OF
YOUR MIND & BODY

"The biggest enemy of good is perfect."

- Voltaire, philosopher

Imagine that you were the best athlete or performer in your area at six years old. Think about what your coaches and instructors might have told you about your body; you were likely given very specific instructions on exactly how to move your body correctly and how to properly position yourself throughout practice. Now, imagine that pattern continuing throughout your childhood. Obviously, this feedback is what will shape the individual that you become. Yet, as your brain develops, you may also begin picking up skills independently with incrementally less coaching. Being the best performer in your discipline with years of practice behind you, you are confident and graceful in your movements. By contrast, your teammates, who have had less practice, tend to be clumsier with their bodies, which leads to more injuries, aches, and pains. Additionally, because you are able to outperform your peers, you develop an even deeper passion for your activity. Along the way, you may suffer a small injury; perhaps a broken bone or sprained ankle. When this happens, your family and coaches quickly send you to the local doctor, trainer, and physical therapist. At such a young age you are able to glide right through the rehabilitation process and soon return to all normal activities.

Now, let's fast-forward ten years. You are a high-level Division I collegiate athlete who suffers a similar injury as before. Instantly, your athletic training staff hops into action telling you exactly what you need to do. After a few weeks in the training room with a daily "rehab menu," you are, once again, back to 100% without even skipping a beat. The speed of your recovery builds your confidence and you feel great to be playing. Notice, however, that little personal transformation has occurred.

A few years go by and you are in the last year of college when you suffer a major injury. Maybe you're a college baseball pitcher with big league aspirations, and you throw your arm out, which requires surgery. Such an injury is exactly the type of physical crisis that could threaten everything you had going for you up until that point. This is your Time Zero — going forward, you will never be the same athlete.

Recognizing Opportunity

Throughout my career as a Doctor of Physical Therapy (DPT), I have specialized in sports and elite performance. During my time serving as the Medical and Rehabilitation Coordinator for the St. Louis Cardinals, I discovered that professional athletes who sustained career-threatening injuries usually had careers that went in one of two directions: Following Time Zero, their career trajectories either shot up to extraordinary levels of success or, more commonly, sank relatively quickly to a disappointing end — very rarely did these athletes get back to their pre-injury normal.

In observing high-caliber individuals dealing with physical adversity, it became clear to me that an injury could be seen as a window of opportunity, an inflection point, for a dynamic transformation to occur in both their athletic careers and well beyond. Yet, in order to make that extraordinary transformation from Injured to Elite, once you have acknowledged your current state, you must make that pivotal next step: Take full ownership and responsibility of your mind and body.

The Challenge

But moving forward with that wisdom is an extraordinary challenge, even for world-class athletes. The reason for this is that many of those top-level performers have never been forced to take full control of their own mind and body.

Think about the many star athletes that have had their careers come to an end due to injuries. NBA center Yao Ming, MLB/NFL All-Star Bo Jackson, MLB star pitcher Kerry Wood, and NFL quarterback Andrew Luck are just a few high-profile examples. Quarterback Andrew Luck told reporters that the attempt to overcome a cycle of injuries had "...taken [his] joy of this game away." Bo Jackson, whose NFL career was cut short due to a hip injury in 1991, told *USA Today* in an interview "If I knew back then what I know now, I would have never played football. Never." All of these athletes have had tremendously successful careers, but what separates these individuals from those that overcome injury and retire on different terms? This became a burning question of mine as I worked with MLB baseball players and other elite performers.

Something that kept coming up repeatedly is the sense that the purpose of many of these players to continue to achieve physical success became external — the agenda of their family, agent, team, or even their fans. They lost control of their internal purpose in looking to please others. That is why, in my practice, I challenge clients and patients to get back to their own sense of purpose in life when challenged with physical adversity. It starts by taking ownership of their mind and body.

Fear Itself

Remember your first appointment with a medical or performance professional after the injury. Hopefully, during that first session you were thoroughly assessed. Based on that assessment, were you given information that empowered you to take ownership of your body? Did you request this info?

Speaking as a clinician, I can tell you that often my clients will give up control immediately by asking simply: "So what do I do, Dave? They'll usually preface it by saying things like "You're the expert..." If you are any type of medical professional, I am sure you have encountered this exact scenario countless times.

While to patients, it may appear that great clinicians always have an exact idea of what to do next, the truth is though the best medical professionals do have useful advice to give, most will strive to guide you to becoming your own master. Unfortunately, in many situations, the hand-holding that occurs when we are young carries over into our adult lives, and this can hinder our overall performance. This is why you must, from the beginning, be mindful of falling into the trap of overreliance on medical professionals.

Frequently, patients over-rely on clinicians because the fear of the unknown becomes as difficult for patients as the injury itself. The good news is, there exists a way for individuals to build a personal road map towards self-ownership and recovery.

Building Your Road Map

So what are the first steps to building your map? It may seem impossible now, but let me tell you a story:

Uri Levine, co-founder of mapping application Waze, which was acquired by Google for almost a billion dollars in 2013, created the first prototype of the app in Tel Aviv with a blank page for a map. On the "Tony Robbins Podcast" (10/7/2019), Uri stated: "When the first driver drove, we collected the GPS data from the device and when we drew this GPS data on the blank page, we got to see something like the route this driver travelled. And when we started to get this data from a lot of drivers, we started to figure out this is starting to look like a map, and if there is a lot of density then we figured out that this is a highway versus a street and if this is an intersection where no one is making a left turn, then this is an intersection where no left turn is allowed, and if there is a road where 100 people are going in one direction, and zero in the other direction, then this is a one-way street. When we started to have more and more drivers then we can generate the traffic information and help people avoid that." If the average person would have tried the Waze app at that time, they would have hated it, but that didn't stop the Waze team who continued to add data points consistently improving their product. Waze wasn't (and still isn't) perfect, but that didn't stop Levine.

These same principles hold true for our own mind and body when it comes to navigating physical challenges. Those initial tests and assessments mentioned in the previous section might give us some valuable information, but they aren't perfect. It is our job to continue adding data points to our road map in order to try and avoid the unforeseen traffic jams with our recovery. You have to keep in mind: There is no one piece of information or level of assistance that will take you fully to your destination. That is why I encourage my clients early on to take ownership of their situation by metaphorically taking the driver's seat in their rehabilitation process.

Just as Waze gives users suggestions for their route based on data points from other users, you are going to gather personal data points to plot the route to your recovery, and beyond. Doing this will show you the best path forward, instead of one that might be better for another individual or "driver." Additionally, similar to how Waze depends on a driver's exact time and location, your best path forward will rely on constantly identifying where you are, or your unique set of circumstances at that moment.

For example, perhaps your body feels great on a particular day, but your mindset is lackluster because of a rough patch in your personal life. Imagine it's 5:30pm, and you walk into the clinic or training room after an intense argument with your significant other, and then your clinician asks you to perform a really hard new exercise. How would that make you feel? Do you think the added stress around your relationship might affect your rehabilitation that day? In this situation, the clinician, who doesn't know about the argument, would be forced to take your struggle and frustration with the exercise at face value and provide you with faulty data points based on their assessment. Being in control here would mean giving them a general sense of your state of mind so they can adjust your treatment. That way you are both moving forward with a shared sense of your progress, and adding useful data points to your map.

I've talked about data points generally up to this point, but you may be wondering exactly what I mean. Rest assured that this isn't going to require reading through a *Gray's Anatomy* textbook, or getting your PhD in Psychology. Instead, building your own map will involve developing the ability to self-assess and monitor both your mind and body.

Learning the Language

Movement is the language the mind speaks to the body. While the mind communicates in electrical signals rather than words, the process does begin with a level of positive self-talk. For the patient, an example of this positive self-talk would include affirming thoughts such as that you are an able-bodied person. More specifically, if you're that baseball player who blew out his arm from earlier in the chapter and you are coming out of your elbow brace for the first time since surgery, moving your arm must involve the belief that the arm is actually safe to move. Though our level of confidence can be influenced by our medical professional's suggestions — for instance, if your surgeon instructed you that it is okay to start moving your elbow — ultimately, you are the one who needs to manifest a mindset of faith in your body's ability to heal; you are in charge of your decisions.

Interestingly, the same part of the brain responsible for

decision-making (the prefrontal cortex) is also the part of the brain that makes decisions such as whether or not to perform a physical movement or task. Though much of this process is unconscious, in order to restore full function after injury, it is important to consciously own the decision to progress into healing. This helps improve communication from our mind to our body, the experience we call movement.

Starting Slow

Just as Waze learns about new roads and traffic flows, starting to perform certain actions for the first time after an injury will give you the opportunity to collect many "data points" and begin to learn your body's patterns. It is important to give yourself time to learn these patterns as they become integrated into your nervous system. This is why rushing through the early phase after a physical challenge is not wise. In the same way Uri Levine had to allow the early version of Waze to naturally learn the patterns of traffic, you must also be patient to avoid missing out on learning important patterns during the beginning of the rehabilitation process. Think about it: If you make a wrong turn from out of your driveway, it is a whole lot easier to correct then if you turn onto the wrong highway later. Give yourself some leeway early on!

Understanding the data points does mean you must pay attention to your mind and body, what it doesn't mean is that you should obsess over every little data point. Instead of dissecting every symptom and sensation, the focus should be on the big picture patterns in your post-injury recovery. Indeed, part of being an elite-level performer is the ability to know how, when, and what to tune out from what their mind and body tells them. Consider this graph:

Bell Curve of Mind-Body Sensitivity

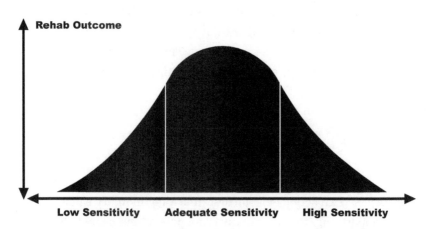

Left side of the curve shows a third of people who show low "Patient Mind-Body Sensitivity", the middle shows middle third of people with moderate sensitivity, and the right side of the graph shows a third of patients that are overly sensitive to their mind-body connection. As illustrated by the y-axis on the left, being hyper-aware doesn't mean you are making better decisions, and might even hinder your path forward with your rehab process. This sometimes creates a situation where a patient over-scrutinizes every detail and does not allow themselves to take action and break the "pain barrier."

Correctly understanding where to put your attention will require intentional practice that will train your mind to communicate better with your body. Here, intentional practice means time devoted to closely focusing on establishing high-quality movement patterns alongside an optimal attitude, and repetitions of exercises. To echo Uri Levine's quote from the beginning of this chapter, you are not seeking perfection here. Instead, the intention is simply to regain control of your body and movement beyond perceived limitations (being afraid to move an arm after surgery, for example), while developing reference points for your path forward.

Steps Towards Ownership

After you're comfortable with the present and know where you're headed, you can continue to advance on the gaps by pushing incrementally past your perceived limits. This intentional and active practice of your mind-body connection will help transform the thoughts you have about your body's abilities, while maximizing the result of your body's physical efforts. There are four concrete steps to successfully take ownership of your mind and body at this stage:

Step #1: Make a conscious decision to get into the driver's seat, with the understanding that your "vehicle" is in good working order, along with trust and faith in your ability to recover.

The modern human has been around for something like 50,000 years. Compare that with 100-150 years or so modern medicine has been around. The point is, people's bodies have been healing long before our healthcare system as we know it. With that knowledge, you need trust in your own body's ability to heal. Think about the last time you suffered a pretty nasty cut...Now think about the last time you watched a superhero heal herself within seconds. In many ways, the human body is just like that superhero, it just takes us a bit longer than in the movies. As you will learn in a later chapter on mindset optimization: "What we think about, we bring about;" so thinking you will heal will actually enhance your ability to do so.

Step #2: Get constructive feedback from medical professionals that empowers *your* process.

Remember all that talk about data points? Instead of asking for definitive answers, ask your providers and professionals what you should be looking for on your own. Ask them what patterns of movement you should be self-evaluating to decide what steps you need to take to help you progress towards returning to your desired activities? What movement tests can you perform easily on your own? The answers to these questions will empower you to break free from the dependency on your provider, and allow you to create the most effective roadmap towards your intended high-performance goals.

Step #3: Use biofeedback (voluntary control of autonomic bodily functions) in order to more objectively self-assess.

While movements might be accompanied by sensations such as pain, discomfort, or ease, an important intentional practice is to shift your focus to the visual quality of your movement. This can be done by watching yourself in a mirror, on video, or asking another individual to give you feedback while observing your movements. The movement itself should become more meaningful than the sensation accompanying it because those sensations are often strongly influenced by a host of mental and emotional factors; remember the feelings involved in the example of arriving at the clinic after an argument with your partner from earlier in the chapter?

To move your rehabilitation forward, utilize visualization to imagine how you want a movement to look and feel in contrast with your current movement quality and sensations. The trick is keeping your focus on where you want to be, while not dismissing where you currently are, and gradually bringing these two realities together. Having that dual conscious awareness of your current state *and* intended goal is a pillar of going from Injured to Elite.

Humans possess, in our brains, a type of nerve cell (neuron) called a mirror neuron which allows us to imitate movements that we observe. I experienced this phenomenon regularly while I worked for the St. Louis Cardinals.

A big part of my job there was to get injured baseball players throwing again. Since their rehabilitation typically involved a specific throwing program I often built, it was my role to carry out the actual throwing with the player. During this process, I tended to unconsciously imitate the arm movement, or "arm action" as we call it in baseball, of the players I threw with. It was notable that my arm action would mimic the player that I was throwing with at the time. When playing catch with a less experienced person, my arm action would feel awkward and poor. This variety of biofeedback can be used to your advantage when looking to improve your own movements instead of relying on verbal cues and commands from others.

You might ask what if I don't know who or what I should imitate? Well, in my practice I have integrated the visualization and imagery of "ideal movements" with my patients. Instead of just telling them that this is what a given movement should look and feel like, I instruct them to focus on the feeling of moving unrestricted before their injury. There have been many clinicians that have researched the effectiveness of mental imagery and rehearsal strategies to improve performance. One of those studies is titled "Effects of self-administered visuo-motor behavioral rehearsal on sport performance of collegiate athletes". (*Journal of Sport Behavior*, 21(2), 206–218.) which found similar self-administered psychological strategies as mental rehearsal to be a good adjunct to physical practice.

Step #4: Use movement to influence your mental state.

The importance of the mind-body connection was demonstrated to me during my first Tony Robbins seminar in January of 2019. Tony Robbins, one of the world's leading motivational speakers and coaches, suggested that we had the ability to change our present state using both our focus and our physiology. While Robbins and many others repeat the mantra that "What we focus on, we become," the less intuitive, yet equally crucial point is the power our physiological state has on how we feel. A simple way of understanding this concept is by pretending to mimic the facial expressions of certain emotions and observing how it changes your state of mind. This is just like when an actor gets into character by portraying certain physical attributes that coincide with a certain internal demeanor, you can use the same principle to have an effect on your state of mind.

Using your physiological state to influence your mental state to create a positive feedback loop for your overall physical state is a great strategy to gain momentum in overcoming an injury. Think about when your alarm goes off in the morning on a day when you are just dreading going into work or practice. As you begin to stretch, splash some water on your face, and maybe take a sip of cold water, you start to feel mentally energized and ready for the day. Just those simple physical actions are enough to help you power through your mental challenge.

In summary, taking ownership of your mind and body requires you to:

1. Get into the driver's seat of your rehab and performance process.
2. Learn to assess your own movement.
3. Utilize biofeedback, specifically through imagery and visualization of optimal movement.
4. Manipulate your physical state to alter your mindset and regulate your emotions.

Taking the driver's seat requires willpower and a conscious decision to act. Learning how to better self-assess requires you to have empowering conversations with professionals in order to better build a Waze-like personal road map, starting from scratch with no data points.

In this next chapter, I am going to teach you to better integrate the information you receive from medical professionals starting with your first interactions at Time Zero.

CHAPTER 3
CONVERSATIONS WITH PROFESSIONALS

I was 19 years old in my 2nd semester of college at Nassau Community College in Long Island, New York. After getting rear-ended by a car and experiencing some back pain, I was advised to go see the local orthopedist. I remember sitting on the treatment table when a burly hunched-over grey-haired man wearing a white coat walked into the room. After making some friendly small talk, he pointed to an x-ray that they had taken of my spine and said "Ah, see you have some curvature and some spasms here, and here."

The orthopedist then recommended that I do a course of physical therapy, and because a few people suggested that it would be beneficial for me to do this to prevent my back from worsening, I obliged. At the time, I didn't truly believe I needed physical therapy but figured they knew better than me — and I certainly didn't want to end up hunched-over like the doctor himself! So, I went to a few physical therapy sessions where they put some hot packs on me, treated me with some electrical stimulation (which felt like bugs running around on my skin), and walked me through some very basic exercises on a few machines.

Though I was not impressed with the process, I was already, at that age, developing a deep passion for exercise. For that reason, I enjoyed the sessions since they let me see a different form of workout. That said, I quickly realized that I didn't really need to be in that clinic, and that made me somewhat hesitant during future conversations with both healthcare professionals and others about my body. Fast forward to now, I became a clinician myself in a large part to provide others with a better experience than I had at that time.

If you are reading this book, you have probably found yourself having many similar conversations with medical professionals. My goal is to help you improve upon them. This chapter, then, is what I would have told 19-year-old David before he went to that appointment with the burly orthopedist.

Ask Good and Appropriate Questions

Don't be the patient that says: "Doc, just tell me what to do..." Instead, you should ask for information to empower yourself to make decisions about your healing process. Framing questions around the clinician's experience is always a good starting point; pretend to be the doctor for just a moment and consider the difference in how you might answer the following questions:

1. "Is there something wrong with the x-rays of my spine?"
2. "In your experience with patients like me, do most people get back to all normal activities following being rear-ended in an accident with findings on an x-ray like this?"

The first question does not give the clinician an opportunity to see you as an individual and truly help you on *your* path forward. Instead, it sets up a situation where the doctor is free to look at the x-ray in a general way and give a vague and simple answer. She might say: "No, everything looks fine," even though your back still hurts, or "...Well, I see you have some scoliosis here," without giving you any actionable steps to take moving forward. If you keep the focus on the experience of the clinician from their work treating a large number of other individuals with similar patterns of findings, it encourages both of you to keep the bigger picture in mind.

But David, you might be thinking, what's wrong with being told the findings of some specific test or measure? Simple, it's because one specific test or measure rarely tells the full story. Imaging, for example, is just an illustration of shadows that lay beneath the skin, and has limited capability to depict underlying issues especially when it comes to a holistic view of the body. In fact, there are specific cases when performing imaging is required by insurance before they are willing to reimburse the clinician for certain procedures to be performed. Unfortunately, this can skew their clinical decision-making. This is yet another reason why you must be the one in control, and work with people you trust.

The questions you ask should be specific enough to get a clear answer, but still allow for a meaningful discussion. Providing them with useful details may help towards this purpose; asking when you can return to playing a sport, for example, might depend on the position you play. In Major League Baseball all 30 teams have a variety of staff focusing on determining a player's rehabilitation plan and return-to-play progression. This progression is highly scrutinized by an aggregate of knowledge in a multi-disciplinary performance department. A player asking the team physician when they can get back to playing is likely to be given a long-winded answer along the lines of "...We'll get you into rehab, build you a throwing program with the rehab coordinator, followed by a mound progression, and eventually a game progression." Naturally, the player will be closely monitored the whole way.

Not everyone has the luxury of their own organizational rehabilitation coordinator, but you can become your own if you ask the right questions. When I rehabilitated players with the St. Louis Cardinals, I would ask our team physicians questions along the lines of "How long would you recommend a period of no throwing for this pitcher before we begin a light stepwise throwing program?" Even if you aren't familiar with baseball jargon, you can guess that I wasn't looking for a black and white answer, but was using questions like this as a jumping-off point to understand the specific complexities and steps of each player's injury and healing — the "why" was just as important as the "when." For your own injury, you can ask for an estimated return date, but really aim for answers that teach you what steps to accomplish first, and why.

Indeed, though a return date ("you can play again on October 4th") may have a feeling of being specific, it is really quite a subjective answer since so much can happen in the course of rehabilitation. This is why physical therapists, who often spend more time with individual patients than physicians, tend to focus on making and building the progression into a more inclusive process. Still, you are the one making the final call, and asking good questions is the way you build your knowledge base and mental model of the treatment process. The more you know (for this you depend on the experience of your medical professionals along with your own research), the more empowered you will be as a patient and athlete to figure out your own safe and effective program. If all of that still seems unclear, don't worry, we will dive much deeper into this in the load management chapter.

Listen to Your Inner Skeptic

Human Performance is not always an exact science, there are countless clinicians who might all give different assessments of your physical and mental state. For that reason, when a patient asks for my opinion on whether to have surgery versus non-operative management, I always make sure that they have received at least a 2nd opinion. If that 2nd opinion differs from their first professional's opinion, I step in and refer them to a 3rd provider to break the tie. Because invasive measures are being considered this is, of course, a more extreme example. However, the opinion of the professional isn't always the most important one.

Every professional, even the most prestigious, have biases that affect how they might perceive your unique situation. Sometimes those biases are internal, sometimes they're borne from external circumstances. The orthopedist I saw at 19 years-old was likely biased by the fact that he had a business interest in the physical therapy clinic that just so happened to be located below his office. This is called a Physician-Owned Physical Therapy Service, better known as a "POPTS". POPTS have created quite the stir over the past few decades and have even been banned in some states due to the obvious potential conflict-of-interest with referring providers. Since many insurance companies require a prescription and referral to pay for physical therapy services beyond a set amount of care that might be provided through "direct access" to a physical therapist, many physical therapists have argued that there is a conflict-of-interest in a physician self-referring to their own business. However, this still routinely happens. This is not a book about the politics of healthcare, and so I will not provide my opinion on the ethics of POPTS. I am only including them here to give you just one example, unknown to many patients, of an external bias a physician may hold.

Going back to the past me with the information I have now, I would have encouraged myself to engage in a little skepticism, which would have possibly influenced me to seek out a different physical therapy clinic. One that would have given me a more individualized program.

Perhaps you were referred to a top surgeon who recommended a cutting-edge procedure, only to find out that they also had an ongoing research study to prove that treatment's effectiveness. This fact in itself doesn't have to be a deal-breaker but it should hold some weight in your overall decision-making.

Bias or not, the most important information to receive from a medical professional is:

- That the worst part of the injury is likely over.
- That it is safe to move forward.
- Suggested guidelines on the process to do that.

Know the Three Elements of Evidence-Based Practice

Evidence-based practice is defined as the use of evidence to make the best decisions related to patient care. The three elements of this are:

1. What the research shows.
2. What the clinician's experience provides.
3. What the patient's experience provides.

All too often, as clinicians or patients, we emphasize one of these elements and leave the others in the background. It can be a challenge, but the reality is that all three need to be factored into making good decisions for one's health and performance. Going back to my earlier example, even though the research in medical journals related to physical therapy might show little statistically significant benefits for the outcomes of patients receiving physical therapy for back pain, as an avid athlete and exerciser with people around me recommending physical therapy, I was primed to try it despite a lack of research to prove its effectiveness. You must always be asking yourself, "Am I missing something here?" And you can use the elements of evidence-based research as a guide.

Finally, imagine if your referring physician does not have much belief in the effectiveness of physical therapy, simply telling you to try it for a few sessions, and if it doesn't work to come back and make another appointment with her. Do you think the doctor's lack of enthusiasm could impact your perceived effectiveness of the treatment you get? Always examine the beliefs of the clinician, patient, and research outcomes when making important medical decisions. If 19 year-old David knew then that it wasn't as simple as "just do what the doctor says…" perhaps he would have thought more about his other possible options at the time.

Note Specific Keywords

Here's a piece of dead-simple but extremely useful advice: Go into your doctor's appointments with a notebook or your mobile phone ready and when something doesn't sound familiar, write it down! Don't just assume you will remember the word or phrase later or that it will somehow magically come to you. Keep in mind that students of the health sciences undergo years of study to remember and understand medical terminology; even doctoral students become very used to hearing their professors say: "Look it Up!"

Part of empowering yourself during these conversations with medical professionals means, at the very least, increasing your medical and performance vocabulary. While you certainly won't be healed in a 5-minute interaction, you might be exposed to lingo that will give you some insight into the clinical picture of your situation. Writing things down on paper or in your mobile device can also pay dividends when you are aimlessly searching online for the same answers from questionable sources of information. When something sounds Latin, has a lot of syllables, and might end in -itis, (the suffix for a pathology that includes inflammation such as arthritis), cue yourself to mark this as a keyword.

Another piece of advice: Whenever you are in doubt, ask questions! If you're not clear about what the clinician said, ask for clarification! Even if you are already at home and realize you still have questions, don't hesitate to pick up the phone or send an email to the doctor's office. This is your health we're talking about, and caring about it is the doctor's main job. It is not the time to be shy.

Identifying Good Information

Information literacy is defined by the Framework for Information Literacy for Higher Education as "...the set of integrated abilities encompassing the reflective discovery of information, the understanding of how information is produced and valued, and the use of information in creating new knowledge and participating ethically in communities of learning." Or in layman's terms: Information literacy is our ability to, for example, see a piece of information on a website and determine whether it's any good. While it is the expectation that the professionals I mentioned in the sections above are credible sources, the same expectation doesn't extend to the web, where anyone can put up a website pretending to be an expert. Even so, I understand that many patients regularly seek a second opinion from "Dr. Google," so in order to help you make the most out of that research, here is a four-part crash-course on information literacy in sports medicine and performance in order to help you make better decisions on your journey.

#1: Consider the source of information: Who are they, and what is their intention? Are they valid and reliable, or just highly marketed?

Always consider the intent of the information you are receiving. When humans convey information, there is almost always an underlying message, or subtext. Sometimes the intention of the underlying message of information is to persuade you to some action rather than to provide you with unbiased content.

Being persuasive or selling a product are not bad things in themselves — experts should feel confident in marketing their philosophies, after all, but it is also important for patients to understand that talking a good game does not guarantee adherence to strict medical standards.

The underlying message of some content might be influenced by the author's polarizing viewpoint on a topic. In those situations, don't expect them to seriously or fairly consider alternate points-of-view. They may mislead, bend the truth, or outright lie, using their platform to push their opinion instead of helping patients. When you are reading articles, watching social media, and reading books, be wary of the author's agenda. One way to quickly identify a biased author is if they present one viewpoint as absolutely amazing while giving strangely short shrift, or being unduly negative, about others. This will become easier and easier to spot once you've done enough research to have a good overview of a topic.

As mentioned earlier, individual pieces of information alone are not enough to determine the best course of action to get past your injury. Many data points are needed in order to make correlations or to draw even slight conclusions. As you might recall from the statistics section of your math classes, when there is a strong relationship between points, we call this statistical significance. As medical professionals, many of us look for these patterns within our patients. Instead of just relying on tell-tale signs of pathology, we aggregate potential findings to look for sources of dysfunction. This is known as "differential diagnosis."

To summarize, avoid relying on single pieces of information to draw general conclusions about how you should be implementing your program. Make sure to aggregate your findings, whether it's conversations with doctors, online research, or talks with friends or family who have had similar experiences. Your body initially does most of the recovery by itself after any type of trauma, so rushing into making decisions can be counterproductive. Be patient, maintain that open-minded skepticism, and be on the alert for biases when figuring out your first steps. Chances are low that you are going to outsmart the human body which has been evolving to recover from trauma since the beginning of humanity.

#2: Avoid misinterpreting information

Besides the biases of information sources, we also have our own strong biases when interpreting outside sources of information; our past experiences and expectations will heavily influence the information we seek and receive. This is neither good nor bad, it's simply an accepted fact. After all, there's a reason one of the three pillars of evidenced-based practice is the individual patient's experience.

Think of the last self-help Instagram (or other social media) post you saw. What was the content suggesting you do? How might someone else with a different perspective have perceived that content? How would you have perceived it if the look and/or sound of the post was slightly tweaked? Reflecting on this will give you a third-person perspective which will allow you to examine your own biases with a more critical eye.

Another angle to consider is whether you are using a piece of information in a constructive way or a destructive way. An example of a constructive use of the information is simply learning a new perspective on a topic related to your rehabilitation. Whereas destructive uses of the information would be obsessively comparing yourself to others, or hooking onto information as a way to try and cheat your way through the healing process. One thing my years of clinical experience have taught me is that there are no secret healing shortcuts that doctors are keeping from you; attempting to outsmart your body or cheating your way through rehab only catches up with you in the long run.

To make this point more vivid, here is an example: If you broke a bone and looked up bone healing online, you might find, let's say, a social media post or article with the title "Vitamin D Supplementation Improves Bone Health." You love drinking milk, which is often fortified with Vitamin D, and so you might interpret this article to mean that you should be drinking loads of milk. Unfortunately, this advice might be very far from the truth, especially if you are not vitamin D deficient. Looking into the topic deeper, you would discover that there are plenty of sources indicating that dairy is not well-digested by humans, and potentially inflammatory. While this is a fairly benign example — drinking more milk probably won't help you heal any faster, but it's unlikely to harm you — the dozens of fad diets that have come up over the past several decades are examples of misinformation with potentially harmful consequences. They are also an example of how we in society can fall into the trap of misinterpreting information that sounds nice initially, but turns out to be dangerous in the end.

Neither reading this section, nor this whole book can make you an expert in sports medicine and performance. That's not my intention. What I do want to do is begin to empower you to use critical thinking when you encounter concepts and ideas in conversation with medical professionals, friends and family, and in your online research. Really, I urge you to think critically about any information related to rehab and performance exercises, treatment techniques, training styles, recovery tools, nutritional recommendations, mental performance, and the vast array of other elements related to your recovery.

#3: Don't be taken in by how something looks and feels

This does not mean discredit things just because they are well-designed, and certainly does not mean that an idea needs to have iron-clad empirical research behind it to be valid (though it doesn't hurt). What you're looking for is a level of reasoning and rationale behind the concept that you're comfortable with; even if it isn't strictly backed by research, as long it hasn't been repeatedly discredited by studies, an open-minded skeptic would remain uncommitted, maintaining the point-of-view that: Hey, it *could* be true. On the other side of the coin, if something just doesn't make sense to you on some fundamental level, that is a good sign to keep digging into this piece of information. This last point is the crucial one when it comes to flashy social media marketing and attractive, charismatic, personalities peddling the latest in high-performance diets, pills, exercise regimens, etc. Sure, they *might* be effective, but it will never be because the person selling it is hot, or spent a mess of money on marketing.

#4: Is it backed by peer-reviewed research?

Though as I mentioned above, a piece of information can be true even if it's not backed up by research, seeing a result repeated in numerous peer-reviewed studies is still the gold standard when it comes to credibility. The nice thing is that you do not need to have a PhD in order to critically evaluate scientific information in academic journals. As allied healthcare and performance professionals, we use websites such as PubMed (pubmed.gov) in order to perform a simple literature[1] review of a topic. For example, if you are wondering whether working out with kettlebells would be effective for your rehab, use this search strategy to kick-off your research: A simple PubMed search of "kettlebells rehab" brings up several hits including an article published in the *North American Journal of Sports Physical Therapy*, titled "Incorporating kettlebells into a lower extremity sports rehabilitation program".[2] In the abstract (summary) of the article, the last sentence states: "This clinical suggestion outlines the clinical rationale for the inclusion of kettlebell exercises when rehabilitating an athlete with a lower extremity injury." The article does not perform an experiment in order to determine the effectiveness of using kettlebells. Instead, it explains the clinical reasoning (or rationale), along with suggestions for, using kettlebells in a rehab program. These suggestions may be more

---

1   When I write literature here, I'm referring to medical journals, not Charles Dickens.
2   Brumitt, J., En Gilpin, H., Brunette, M., & Meira, E. P. (2010). Incorporating kettlebells into a lower extremity sports rehabilitation program. *North American journal of sports physical therapy* : NAJSPT, 5(4), 257-265.

academically sound then what you read on a social media post, hear on sports radio, or see in the gym. Even so, because the authors didn't actually perform a study, they can offer no evidence for why their advice should be followed. In fact, doing further research, one would discover an article (Meigh et al, 2019)[3] reviewing existing kettlebell studies, actual experiments, that concludes, "The strength of recommendation for kettlebell training improving measures of physical function is weak, based on the current body of literature." This example tells us that just because an article is published in a peer-reviewed journal doesn't make it gospel; there is high-quality as well as low-quality research being published every day. There *is* still value in reading and evaluating academic literature on health because it means that you are raising your level of awareness outside of the traditional channels you may be more accustomed to. Personally, I am still using kettlebells due to a high level of anecdotal evidence based on my personal experience as a clinician (one of the pillars of evidence-based practice). In my opinion, the shape of the kettlebell allows for manipulating the load in many different ways to train the body effectively. However, making larger and more general claims without any evidence, like that kettlebells are the absolute best way to rehab a strained muscle, would certainly affect my credibility with patients and other clinicians.

As a non-professional, you should now be able to critically evaluate a piece of information you receive and understand if there may exist some scientific evidence in its effectiveness. This might just provide a free abstract summary of the article however this gives you more powerful information over a simple video you might have seen through a social media post that likely was not critically studied and published in a research journal. Peer-reviewed journals evaluate all published papers through a network of several expert reviewers prior to being published by the scientific journal. This gives you a starting point to use the same strategies the professionals use to be a better judge of what you see, hear, and read. By no means is this a full course on how to perform and evaluate research, but rather just a way to critique some

---

3   Meigh, N. J., Keogh, J., Schram, B., & Hing, W. A. (2019). Kettlebell training in clinical practice: a scoping review. *BMC sports science, medicine & rehabilitation*, 11, 19. https://doi.org/10.1186/s13102-019-0130-z

of the questions you might have related to your journey from *Injured to Elite*.

"Doctor" is Just a Title

In every situation a practitioner's biases may impact the recommendations and treatment that you receive. Remember that one of the three major elements of evidence-based medicine is the provider's own experiences. The important thing to note here is that, like we discussed in chapter 2, you are always in the driver's seat. When you feel that the practitioner isn't including you in the decision-making process, then it is time to be very skeptical.

Another concept to keep in mind is how a physician's biases might impact the prognosis you are given; many of us clinicians hear athletes tell us "...the doctor told me I will never play again." Yet, somehow the odds are defied and the unthinkable happens — they get back to the game! Whenever you receive negative absolute statements such as "this will *never* occur," or "you *must* do this," be skeptical. Despite their years of training, doctors can't possibly know every potentiality of how a dynamic living being will evolve for the rest of their lives. Thankfully, that is your special story.

Yes, your doctor might be one of the best in the business. Yes, they probably have a great medical education. But what they do not have is a crystal ball, and they are not a force higher than you. The ultimate healer is not your doctor, but you yourself. Don't forget this when you are talking to the experts.

Finally, be aware and maintain a critical eye when doing research online. While the world wide web is amazing, putting a vast amount of medical information in front of you with every search, it is also full of dangerous false information. Be on-guard when you read things that are too good to be true, and treat everything you see with skepticism. If you do find interesting and useful information, don't be afraid to discuss it with a medical professional, whether it be your surgeon, physical therapist, or other member of your performance team. Speaking of performance team, that's what we're covering next!

CHAPTER 4
BUILDING YOUR
PERFORMANCE TEAM

Now that you have decided to take responsibility for your own mind and body and learned how to better navigate conversations with professionals, let's spend some time on the people with whom you'll be having these conversations — your performance team. In this age of social media, we have never been inundated with more options for who to listen to, trust, and follow, and, more importantly, who to work with on our journey towards becoming the best version of ourselves as an athlete and an individual. This chapter is designed to help you develop better habits when it comes to selecting your advisors, paying for their services effectively, and better integrating a "team" into your daily life.

Since at least 2010, the field of sports science and performance management has been instrumental in the widespread development of performance departments within professional and collegiate sports organizations. The missions of these departments are to track and enhance the physical performance of their players while better managing the player's injuries. Over the past five years, these departments have also exponentially grown in Major League Baseball. When I started my career with the St. Louis Cardinals in 2015, I was one of two physical therapists within the organization. Just after my first year, the organization hired a Director of Performance in order to oversee all areas related to player health and performance including strength and conditioning, rehabilitation, athletic training, and sports science. Two years later, I was one of five physical therapists, not counting my assistant, Frankie D'Aversa, who I hired as the Assistant Rehab and Medical Coordinator, but who had the credentials of

Physical Therapist Assistant. Just as many sports organizations have implemented robust performance teams, it is important for every athlete and individual whether an amateur or professional, to have their own strong performance team. You must be the director of your own performance department.

Think about a boxer walking to the ring before a fight. While their music is blasting in the background, they lead a team that will help them during the fight. Imagine if that team was an entourage of 50 people! How would this fighter effectively connect with each of these team members? What if there was conflict between members of the team? Consider the amount of money each of these team members would expect from this fighter. Most importantly for our purposes, how would he manage input from all of those associates? The answers to these questions are the everyday struggles of an up-and-coming athlete, and though it's not unlike a regular workplace where a clear reporting structure and healthy communication reign supreme, what's at stake for an athlete is much higher since her body is her livelihood.

In general, it's best to avoid the confusion of a huge team; the team you build to support your efforts should follow the principle that less can be more. I have found that with too many experts in the training room, their various points-of-view overshadows the performer. With fewer people, you have more control of choosing the right ones. And since building a good rapport with the people on your team should always be the priority, you can spend your time building trust rather than managing conflict. In my own career, not every patient or athlete I have worked with has been an ideal fit. This is something that bothered me early on, but over time I learned that it serves both parties better when those feelings were brought out into the open. Sometimes it meant we parted ways, but just as often it created a stronger relationship through adjustments by one or both parties. Make sure to have a strong and trusting relationship with whomever you decide to be your assistant director (or whatever title you want to use) of performance.

In general, you should look beyond an expert's social media claims or testimonials from high-level athletes as oftentimes these are just a marketing mastermind's illusions. While those things can be data points in your research, you should also ask around to see what others have to say about this potential advisor — both colleagues and clients. Keep in mind, however, that the dynamic of your working relationship with this advisor will not necessarily be the same as for others. I have personally had great working relationships with many Major League Baseball players that my colleagues couldn't stand, and the other way around. So, whatever else you do, definitely pay attention to how the two of you get along. If you get a sense, even just a slight one, that something is off, consider whether this person is truly the one that will get the best out of you.

Recall the three pillars of evidence-based practice you learned in chapter three: The research, experience of the clinician, and experience of the patient. Note that two of those are you and your expert advisor. So then how does one determine if they are on the same wavelength as their advisor? It should feel as though a conversation can flow naturally in both directions with relative ease. This doesn't mean that the two of you need to agree on everything, or that they should carry out your every request. Instead, your conversations should feel like discussions rather than receiving orders. As I mentioned before, if this doesn't exist early on, it can still be achieved through a soft confrontation; do not be afraid to voice concerns you may have with the way your advisor is communicating. Think of this as having a professional meeting with a colleague instead of an intimidating "Doctor-Patient Relationship."

This type of conversation has happened several times in my own career. When athletes and patients of mine have confronted me, it has almost always led to improved rapport and not a breakdown of the relationship. Approaching the situation with good faith prevents a confrontation from negatively affecting the relationship in the long run. In the worst-case scenario, the clinician should be able to refer you to someone else. Either way, this is all part of a normal clinician/client working partnership.

Below is a description of the skillsets you should look for when building your own performance team in addition to your treating physician. While you may not require each of these professionals,

having some combination of the skills below within even just a few of
your advisors can be an extraordinary advantage in your journey from
injured to elite.

The Medical and Rehabilitation Expert

This person can be a physical therapist, athletic trainer, surgical
orthopaedist, chiropractor, naturopathic doctor, osteopathic medical
doctor, osteopathic therapist, or primary care sports medicine doctor.
They should have both academic and hands-on experience managing
physical injuries, conditions, and illnesses that are similar to yours.
Since your body's physiology plays a large part of the healing process,
understanding medical physiology at a high-level should be, at least,
part of their background.

Throughout the rehabilitation process this professional should
be well equipped at understanding the many other systems of your
body which can be impacted by injury, and affect overall healing. For
example, an understanding of the cardiovascular and integumentary
(skin) systems is useful since they are areas that may need to be closely
monitored post-injury. Inspecting the healing of a wound after an
injury or surgery requires an understanding of infectious red flags, and
changes in circulation after injury might require performing different
physical tests.

A few of my patients who have undergone minimally invasive
orthopedic surgery (arthroscopy), have suffered from a blood clot
(known as a Deep Vein Thrombosis) shortly after surgery that became
a medical emergency. Knowledge of how to properly deal with these
situations requires more than just understanding principles of
rehabilitation. These are just a couple of reasons why a combination of
expertise in rehabilitation guidelines and understanding what medical
red flags to look for will be very valuable to exist in one person.

In addition, he or she must possess a deep understanding of
your goals and individualized needs. If you are a baseball player, and
this person has never picked up a baseball, make sure that they have

the specialized knowledge they need to help you properly. This is where asking targeted questions comes in handy during your interactions with this professional. The medical and rehabilitation expert should also understand the importance of a holistic approach to rehabilitation which includes a combination of exercise, hands-on work, education, and mental approaches. This journey is a process that is not always linear. Having the right expert to help you build a written or visual progression can be one of the most important steps forward.

The Strength and Conditioning Expert

To ensure a seamless transition between rehab and performance, this person should be working in tandem with the rehab & medical expert to advise you on organizing a more intensive training program on top of your rehabilitation. Don't wait to start this process; for example, if you have a shoulder injury, your strength and conditioning expert might recommend that you utilize a weighted vest and train the lower body with squats and lunges even during the first week after injury. This keeps stress off the shoulder, while still loading the lower half of the body — it allows you to maximize your training during a time that might otherwise be wasted.

Training the rest of an athlete's body after injury has been investigated in an article by Drs. Dan Lorenz and Michael Reiman[4]. Published in 2011, their paper details evidence in support of the use of strength and conditioning principles while in the physical rehabilitation setting of athletes. Although the subject lacked high-level studies at the time the article was published, in this preliminary report, the authors outline training guidelines throughout the different phases of rehabilitation. Early on they recommend training the joints above and below the injured area while working on low intensity endurance exercises of stabilizing muscles. As the athlete progresses with their rehabilitation, more intensive strength and speed training are initiated. Although a point of common sense, the article states "Communication

---

4   Lorenz, Dan & Reiman, Michael (2011) "Integration of Strength and Conditioning Principles into a Rehabilitation Program" *International Journal of Sports Physical Therapy* 6(3): 241-53.

and collaboration amongst all individuals caring for the athlete is a must." When this is achieved, good decisions are usually made. In my own work, I've noticed that strength and conditioning early on after injury, when safely implemented, can improve the moral of an athlete, and even help optimize their recovery process.

Working with this person on your strength and conditioning program will help you focus on the function you do have, rather than obsessing over your limitations, and the pain that may accompany it. This motivation gives the body fuel to propel itself forward and become more resilient in a period of physical distress as it adapts to the demands imposed on it over time. On the other hand, constantly poking and prodding at the healing parts of your body with exercises and movements can overwork those areas and even agitate the healing process.

Keep in mind that your strength and conditioning coach can be the same person as your medical and rehab expert as long as strength and conditioning is an area of their expertise and ongoing experience. The common credential for collegiate or professional strength and conditioning coaches is a Certified Strength and Conditioning Specialist (CSCS). If you see these credentials near their name then that is a good starting point. Learn more at https://www.nsca.com/certification/cscs/.

The Mental Performance Expert

The mental performance expert here is defined as a person with expertise in a combination of psychology and sports performance. There's no requirement that they be a licensed psychologist — if you know a life coach that is helpful in keeping your mind right, go for it. Of course, this expert can also be any combination of the aforementioned professionals, as long as they have the appropriate knowledge and skills.

Whoever you choose, it is extremely important that they are able to give you some level of advice related to your mental and emotional wellbeing. Not being able to do what you love, what you've spent so much time doing, can cause psychological stress that extends to other areas of your life. Having a mental performance expert in your corner can help keep some of those negative feelings in check and lead to a better overall mental state and mindset, assisting with developing your life goals and challenges during this period of physical crisis.

Keep in mind that a weekly or monthly video-chat or phone conversation with this individual can be as effective as physically going to a therapist's office, so you needn't worry if you don't have someone readily available in your local area.

To give you a sense of what a mental performance expert might look like, I am one of the first physical therapists to apply for an advanced certification as a Certified Mental Performance Consultant (CMPC) through the Association for Applied Sports Psychology. The following website can easily help you find a referral to a CMPC-credentialed clinician. These individuals can serve as a great resource during the physical rehabilitation process for any athlete. For more information, check out: https://appliedsportpsych.org/certification/cmpc-directory/

The Sport-Specific Skill Expert

Remember that your journey has a destination! A destination that probably involves a high-level of a specific physical skill. Whether it is getting back to an elite level of organized athletics, conquering ultramarathons, or simply recreational golf, the Injured to Elite process is designed to highlight your rehabilitation as a reset point and an opportunity in order to perfect your skills. Since you are not engaging in full-on practice or competition and have more time in your schedule, perhaps you have some time to perform intentional and blocked practice sessions for sports-specific skill development. Your sports-specific skill expert is the go-to person for this. They must be a specialist at your sport or activity (consider whether you need to go even deeper to look for someone with expertise in a particular position, even), and more importantly, be very effective at giving you actionable feedback in order to improve your skills. As with all of these experts, it needs to be a person with whom you can communicate freely; someone who takes the time to get in-depth and explain themselves, while at the same time being able to listen closely and understand your needs. Most vitally, this individual should be respectful of your individualized needs based on your physical and mental state after injury. Every team member must be open to working as a team.

Making Your Team Work For you

Your time is precious. To use it wisely, I recommend getting comfortable working remotely with your team. While initially, it can be good to build rapport with face-to-face interactions, eventually remote and virtual engagement can free up time and money while forcing you to take a more active role in the process (recall what I talked about in chapter two). Video chat, phone calls, videos, text messages, specialized mobile apps and even email are all great examples of ways to communicate with your team members. Trust me, you will thank yourself for utilizing this approach as it will encourage you to learn how to master the healing process by more heavily relying on yourself to figure things out, with just enough professional guidance where you truly need it.

In general, try and avoid using friends, family members, or former coaches as team members. When dealing with each other on a professional basis, these relationships can become muddled and make it challenging to stay objective on your journey. While it is not always a deal-breaker, I caution you to try and keep the personal biases to a minimum as the focus needs to be on you.

Please remember that you should remain in the driver's seat with these advisors on your team; your interactions with them should be empowering, helping to fill gaps in your knowledge, rather than developing into dependent relationships. What you are looking for is people to help you with a framework for a return-to-activity program that gives you some structure along with good advice on how to execute the program well.

Last but not least, to become the best director of your performance team, remember the information literacy lessons I taught you in chapter three. Be critical and use them to evaluate the information that is presented to you by the experts on your team. Many people out there are charismatic and talk a good game, but when you dig a little deeper, end up as nothing more than clever salespeople. Don't fall for that. Expertise is important, but, first and foremost, you need to build your team on the basis of trust.

By now I trust that you are an open-minded skeptic in the driver's seat of your healing journey. Now it's time to get to work rehabbing your mindset.

CHAPTER 5
REHABBING YOUR MIND

"I'm reflective only in the sense that I learn to move forward. I reflect with a purpose."

-Kobe Bryant

The Injured to Elite approach is all about a personal transformation to turn a seemingly negative event towards a positive outcome — a process which will serve as an impetus to create immense change physically, mentally, and spiritually, ultimately helping you feel a higher sense of purpose. As has become apparent up to this point, the body is only one aspect of that. Close readers will notice the play on words in this chapter's title, a little fun to show you how much emphasis I put on the role of the mind in the rehabilitation process. Indeed, rehab is defined by the Merriam-Webster Dictionary, as "... the action of restoring something that has been damaged to its former condition." But as we discussed earlier, the human body has natural abilities to heal itself, and tapping into this ability after Time Zero has everything to do with getting your mind and body on the same page. So that definition of rehab, especially the weight people put on its physical aspect, is clearly different from how I see it in this book.

In this chapter, you are going to learn how to overhaul your mindset in order to tap into your fullest potential; you are going to learn about the very strong relationship your body has with your thoughts and emotions, along with the intense connection between fear and pain. We'll start by diving into pain science, then I will introduce you to tools such as the "reset breath," meditation, journaling, and others, and turn you onto concepts such as "thought viruses," the power of momentum, and the centrality of grit in the healing process. As you'll see, the lessons in this chapter are very personal to me; I came to them through special mentors and friends, and by reading life-changing books. Most importantly, these are tools and ideas that got me through incredibly tough times in my life, and I continue to use them every single day.

Back to Time Zero

Let's start by backtracking for a second to your Time Zero event. What is one of your first memories of it? If I had to guess it would likely be a a physical memory of pain or discomfort. Some people actually report going blank because of the intense pain they felt, while others remember every little detail of the day, from the temperature to the face of someone passing by right at that moment of injury. Our nervous system and senses actually heighten our awareness during a fight or flight scenario. This involuntary pathway is part of our sympathetic nervous system, which responds to imminent threat, usually with an emotional state of fear.

Our sympathetic nervous system, which activates when we are in a threatened physiological state, has many functions that share common pathways with our thoughts and deep emotions. Another name for this complex system that deals with deeper emotions and pain is the limbic system. It is this area of our brain that contains the more primitive parts that we have in common with other mammals. Similar to the way the high-tech, sensor-filled cars hitting the roads these days are extremely reactive to threats they perceive on the road, our nervous system is constantly scanning our surroundings for threats and, sometimes incorrectly, reacting.

Most readers will admit that their first memory after injury is related to a sense of fear and pain. In fact, it's predictable because we are simply programmed that way. Just as artificial intelligence systems learn based on previous events, our brains hold tightly onto these memories as a "primitive" solution so we can avoid those situations in the future. For instance, when a child touches a hot stove and gets a little burn, they tend to remember that the stove is hot and are cautious about touching it again. Later, as adults, we learn to control and understand those instinctual feelings so we can, for example, clean the stove without fear, knowing that it is off. The point is that we have the ability to override these previous associations with experiences and feelings via conscious decision-making on the part of our brain, the same area that is responsible for many of our movements.

The Truth About Pain

As someone who encounters the pain of others on a daily basis, you may be surprised when I tell you that pain is not actually a trustworthy indicator of your physiological state. The fact is that your own thoughts and emotions can impact how you perceive pain in any given moment. This makes pain an unreliable, and I would even go as far as to say limiting, guide during the rehab process starting with your Time Zero moment. The memories you've clung to since your Time Zero have likely had a major influence on how you have experienced pain since.

Here's a little crash course on the brain: An area called the thalamus is responsible for sending and integrating pain signals to other areas of the brain. The amygdala is the part of the brain that processes emotions — it has been referred to in the past as the "reptilian brain." Our frontal lobe deals with decision-making and memories. These parts of the brain are all deeply connected within our limbic system, and exactly the areas which we are looking to better control moving forward.

To start, if we improve our emotional state (processed by the amygdala), it can have a profound effect on our perception of pain through the thalamus, an integration center of pain which communicates with the amygdala.

A Quick Exercise

Follow along with this next exercise as you read it:

Take a moment and think of a positive thought related to the benefits this book will bring to your journey towards a better life after your injury or physical crisis. Next, physically act out an emotion such as happiness or excitement by smiling, opening your eyes wide, and breathing a bit deeper. Feel this emotion run through your entire body starting with your face, progressing down into your neck, spine, shoulders, arms, hands, chest, stomach, pelvis, hips, legs, and feet. Now, focus back on your Time Zero and your perceived physical limitations. It's okay to allow your emotions to go back to the pain you have been experiencing and focus on the events that led up to this. How does your body feel now that you have changed your focus from happiness or excitement to the past? Now, take a little time to return to positive feelings about your current and future progress. Bring an intense attention to all of the functions you are beginning to regain and the promise of a better life emanating from your Time Zero to the present moment. Through the exercise, you were able to quickly take control of your emotions in order to instill a physical feeling. And though it may not have been easy at the moment, with practice you will be able to snap into a positive state whenever you need to. The next section will give you a simple tool to help you further develop this ability.

The Reset Breath

The right mindset is a foundational tool for going from injured to elite and conscious breathing is one of the most effective ways to take immediate ownership and control of our physiological and psychological state. I owe major credit to my mentor John Denney (more about him soon) for teaching me the power of the reset breath.

The reset breath is a beautiful, easy, and powerful practice to develop. Truly, you can do it anytime you have a few seconds, but it really works wonders when you have just experienced a setback or difficulty, and/or when you have a challenge ahead of you. Here's how to do it, step-by-step:

Step #1: Start by centering your mind's focus to your heart, John calls this "Heart Mind Focus." Keep this step simple: Focus on your heartbeat and feel your love and passions brewing.

Step #2: Next, take a slow deep breath in through your nose and out of your mouth through pursed lips like you are blowing out a candle. The out-breath should be long and complete.

Step #3: As you complete your breath feel a sense of relaxed energy flow throughout your entire body, all the way to your fingertips and toes. If you have ever practiced any form of eastern martial arts or medicine, you may be familiar with the concept of "chi" or your energy flow. Chi, in Chinese, is synonymous with "breath," and in Sanskrit "Life Force," so think of the reset breath as harvesting your natural energy flow in order to call up your inner reserve when you need it most. You will know that you have completed a good reset breath when you feel a sense of peace flowing throughout your mind and body and you are reinvigorated and ready to face the world.

Step #4: Once you have completed this full, high-quality breath, focus on something for which you are grateful in your life. My advice is to keep it simple and specific. Repeat in your head after this thought, "thank you, thank you, thank you!"

That was the reset breath. Once you've taken a moment to give yourself this gift, go forth and complete whatever task you had ahead of you causing either some sense of performance anxiety or fear. In your state of calm, you should now be able to visualize your intended result. John Denney routinely teaches the reset breath to top PGA tour golfers, who use it to center themselves when they have to perform under tremendous pressure. Naturally, this has produced career-changing results for these golfers!

John Denney

I first met performance coach John Denney in South Florida, when I was working with the St. Louis Cardinals. I was initially introduced to him through one of my clients, an elite kite surfer, and later ran into him by chance at a mall in Palm Beach Gardens. John soon became a friend and mentor to me, teaching me ideas and techniques that have had an enormous impact on my life. Shortly after that chance encounter, I met him at his office in Jupiter and it was there that he shared with me his background and philosophies when it came to elite performance.

During that conversation, John asked me if I meditated. As an open-minded skeptic, I was intrigued, but I admitted that I didn't regularly meditate. He explained that he had put together his own guided meditation program after being challenged by a friend to post a Facebook Live video of himself meditating every day to the Jupiter, Florida sunrise. Since John was looking to become more consistent with his own meditation practice at the time, he followed through for a whole year eventually creating a website for The Harmony Exercise at https://theharmonyexercise.com. At our meeting, John told me with his strong, vigorous voice: "Dave, meditation will change your life."

The Harmony Exercise uses progressive relaxation, along with concepts including health, harmony, gratitude, abundance, and right action, a total of seven life principles. As an avid athlete and elite big wave surfer himself, over time he integrated these principles into his own physical journey.

"Taking Right Action" is the seventh principle of the Harmony Exercise. After going through the first six principles, the guided meditation takes you through the step of right action which informs the meditator to "...take right action having trust and faith that all is working out in perfect order." During this last part of The Harmony Exercise we take those previous positive statements of affirmation and put them into right action. If our goal is to reprogram the thought of perfect health into our belief system (bs), we affirm, "I am perfect health," then in this last step we take a leap of faith into the spiritual side to assure us that all is going to work out on our journey after injury.

This is not a religious book, but one must appreciate the spiritual element to achieve their highest potential. John Denney teaches that "...faith is the connecting link between hoping and knowing." So putting our affirmations into right action can work to bring our hope of recovery into our reality. But it requires being in a state where you are self-regulating your mindset and emotions. When I began practicing The Harmony Exercise, I was often confused about what that right action step may be, but I've grown to realize that right action is a natural process when we put ourselves in the right state of mind and body with the use of specific strategies. Higher forces in nature energize us with momentum to push onward. This likely won't be a surprise to you if you are already spiritually-seeking. Likely you can attest to some level of guidance from higher forces when achieving higher states of mind, body, and spirit. For those not oriented in this direction, I won't tell you what to believe, instead I'll share what science has to say about meditation, my own experiences with it, and down-to-earth tangible steps to get you started.

Meditation is Medication

Meditation is an age-old practice that takes form in different ways through many traditions around the world. In the United States, the rise of mindfulness practices over the past few decades have brought with them a variety of different meditation styles. While meditation has been anecdotally praised by practitioners who make all sorts of claims about its effectiveness, there is also a fair amount of scientific study that supports the benefits of meditation for all sorts of mental and physical conditions. For example, a 2010 article[5] in the journal *Behavioral and Brain Functions* describes a small study that

---

5   Kaul, P., Passafiume, J., Sargent, C. R., & O'Hara, B. F. (2010). Meditation acutely improves psychomotor vigilance, and may decrease sleep need. *Behavioral and brain functions* : BBF, 6, 47. https://doi.org/10.1186/1744-9081-6-47

supports the idea that meditation may decrease the amount of sleep one needs. A 2017 survey article[6] found that in the studies it reviewed, "Mindfulness meditation was associated with statistically significant improvement in depression, physical health-related quality of life, and mental health-related quality of life." Finally, you might be interested to know that an article from the *Journal of Positive Psychology*[7] found that 15 minutes of meditation done by a beginner provides positive feelings that are comparable to a day of vacation! And these are just three of the, literally, hundreds of easily accessible articles on the effects of meditation on helping treat medical problems and to promote general happiness.

On a more personal level, the meditation practice that I have incorporated into my own daily routine has brought me closer to clarifying my vision and achieving my dreams, including writing this very book. Part of my morning routine when writing this book was waking up and performing John Denney's guided Harmony Exercise, then going off to accomplish my goal of writing 500-1000 words per day. Meditating allowed me to organize my thoughts and harness my creativity in ways I wasn't expecting when I first started to do it.

At that time, I was going through something of a professional crises. I had left the Cardinals the year before and moved across the country to Los Angeles. There, I worked with both athletes and the general population at ADI Rehab. Though there was some fulfillment in helping less athletic individuals work through their injuries, I began to question my sense of purpose as it pertained to my profession.

Directly after my time in professional baseball, I had decided that I was going to start a consulting company to oversee the medical and performance needs of professional athletes, mainly baseball players. The idea was to do work similar to what I was doing for the Cardinals, but instead of putting the team first, I would put all my focus

6   Hilton, L., Hempel, S., Ewing, B. A., Apaydin, E., Xenakis, L., Newberry, S., Colaiaco, B., Maher, A. R., Shanman, R. M., Sorbero, M. E., & Maglione, M. A. (2017). Mindfulness Meditation for Chronic Pain: Systematic Review and Meta-analysis. *Annals of behavioral medicine : a publication of the Society of Behavioral Medicine,* 51(2), 199-213. https://doi.org/10.1007/s12160-016-9844-2
7   Christopher J. May, Brian D. Ostafin & Evelien Snippe (2020) The relative impact of 15-minutes of meditation compared to a day of vacation in daily life: An exploratory analysis, *The Journal of Positive Psychology,* 15:2, 278-284, DOI: 10.1080/17439760.2019.1610480

on the athlete, working directly with their agent. It made sense that the world's greatest athletes should have their own consultant to ensure that all of their physical needs are being well met throughout their careers.

I thought it was a good idea but in Los Angeles, I struggled to build the business in my spare time while putting in days at ADI. Although the idea was to leverage my work in professional baseball and sports performance to build a development program in southern California, I found myself questioning everything about the business model; the original inspiration was to better serve athletes without the bias of a team setting but it seemed as though it just wasn't complete. After a while, I knew I had to shift course to work on my own personal and professional development. There was something missing in my plans. This turned out to be my cue to make some serious changes in my own mindset.

Coincidentally, my girlfriend at the time (now my fiancée, who you met in chapter 1) was going through her own professional journey attempting to break into the event-planning industry after quitting a job in recruiting. At around this time, the two of us were consistently listening to personal development audiobooks and podcasts together, working out every day, and eating healthy. To be honest, I was amazed and inspired by Olya's determination — most people wouldn't have the drive to go to event venues all over Los Angeles and personally hand their resume to hiring personnel, but she did. Olya quit her job on a Wednesday and within two short days was hired on-the-spot as a wedding coordinator for a premier floral company, a job that she had been dreaming about for the past five years.

My journey took a bit longer, but slowly I began to share the content I was integrating into my own personal development with patients. Though I was a psychology major during my undergraduate studies, and had always appreciated the psychosocial elements of rehabilitation, I seldomly brought these issues up to patients. Now, however, I was taking the actual steps of working those concepts into my patient-related care.

At first I was hesitant to share this with my patients, but eventually I couldn't help but share The Harmony Exercise with a few patients who were going through a tough time. In a private room, I would set up my laptop and play them a guided meditation. I wasn't surprised when, despite their recent injuries, patients reported feeling a strong sense of calm. It was at those moments that my role shifted from just considering what exercise I prescribed to help increase my patient's mobility to a more holistic view of my patients and their injuries. The big question became: How could I help them transform their patterns of negative thought viruses into actionable steps to take control of their situations? This was the line of thinking that eventually led to the Injured to Elite philosophy, and the book you're reading today.

In a nutshell, this is why meditation is included in this book. Meditation allows you the time to start your day off on the right foot and is a great way to press the reset button every morning. Your journey towards peak performance will have many challenges (including your injury), and it is vital to start each and every day with the concepts of health, gratitude, harmony, and right action. While I'm not going to delve into exactly what type of meditation you should adopt, I am biased by my own positive experiences with The Harmony Exercise and the Headspace app. That said, my main concern is not what app or style of meditation you choose, it is that you do yourself the service of sitting down to meditate. Once you've tried a few methods, you can make a decision as to which you prefer using your own judgement. And if you are already meditating, even better! The important thing here is to use some time out of your day towards clearing your mind and putting yourself in a physiological state of relaxation. In the next chapter, you will learn the importance of this state of relaxation, but before we move on to more mental tools and concepts, I want to get you started with a few basic tenets of meditation that I think are especially useful.

First Things First

Meditate first thing in the morning to start each day with the renewal of your mind. In general, when you are trying to make something a habit, do that thing early in the day rather than allowing for the excuses that will occur throughout the day. The length of time doesn't have to be a day either; you can front-load difficult stuff early in the week, too. A common example of this is putting the workouts that we tend to dread on a Monday rather than later in the week to ensure that we get them done while we are still full of willpower and motivation.

"The more you resist, the more it will persist!"

Learn how to let go of distractions during meditation. For example, if you have a significant other walking around in another room or if there is construction going on next-door, avoid fighting it. Accept the distraction and let your mind move on to other things. This is also a good exercise for those dealing with pain. You can let your mind focus on the distraction for a few moments and then move away from it. It's hard at first, but with practice you'll find that it gets a lot easier.

In the Headspace app, these distraction thoughts are compared to "cars passing by." You hear them as they come, and as they go, but there's no point in fighting them. The distractions around you and in your mind will certainly exist, a simple piece of wisdom in dealing with them is to just remind yourself that they are supposed to exist. Distractions are totally normal.

The Power of Affirmations

One of the most important concepts John Denney shared with me is the use of effective statements of these "I am" affirmations. Part of the Harmony Exercise uses affirmation statements such as "I am perfect health," "I am perfect harmony," and "I am grateful." Whether you are performing the Harmony Exercise or any other version of meditative practice, these positive affirmations can also help reprogram the beliefs you hold related to your performance goals. Affirmation statements can be helpful in your physical life too by shaping your total perception of the controllable elements in your healing journey. Now, let's make this relevant to your post-injury process.

Most conventional rehab situations incorporate a home exercise program and the Injured to Elite method is no different in this regard. As a clinician, when I've asked my patients if they have been doing their exercises, I often heard statements like: "I need to get better at doing them," or "I want to try and spend more time getting them into my day." If you catch yourself making similar statements, it is time to use positive affirmation statements to change your habits.

Repeating these statements during your meditation will eventually help you make the steps recommended in this book into habits. Remember, as John Denney often says: Thoughts are things!

I once called John up when I was hitting a rough patch in the development of my business, and started to drop off with my meditation schedule. I told John, "I am struggling to stay focused." In response, John shouted: "Change your story Dave! You are focused, and you are doing it!"

Your Time Zero has already changed your story from the one you thought you were living in before your injury, but in order to take control, you need to write your story's next chapters, or else outside forces will write them for you. Without regulating your thoughts and changing your belief system, you risk letting the story be written for you rather than by you. Your physical goals will not be achieved for you by your doctor, therapist, or coach, but by you. Meditation is the daily practice by which you will remind yourself of this principle.

Once You Affirm it, Write it!

A little while ago I mentioned my morning routine. One thing it typically involves is meditation and the other is journaling. Taken together, these two activities are a powerful duo when it comes to self-motivation and long-term persistence. But I didn't always journal.

Here's how I started:

One day, I was browsing the Amazon bookstore in Marina Del Rey and saw a black folder-style planner. It was Brendon Burchard's High Performance Planner. I had been looking for a more organized way to record my thoughts on paper. Before, I would spend a lot of time just writing out my ideas for different projects related to my business content — ideas for webinars and other online education — but the different strands of thoughts would get tangled; it was just too disorganized to be usable. After getting the planner, I encouraged myself to sit down every morning and condense all of my thoughts into those moments of writing. Since my time was limited I was forced to be brief, which helped me get to the point faster. Now, every morning I wake up, meditate, and then write down my priorities and goals for the day in the high performance planner.

Having a performance journal (It doesn't matter if it's the high performance planner or a simple notebook) is a tenet of the Injured to Elite philosophy. I believe that everyone in search of high performance after injury should have some form of a journal. Simply writing down your thoughts and priorities is a start but here are a few steps to super-charge your journaling:

Step #1: Write your overall mission and goals each day.

Keep your rehab and performance mission statement 1-2 sentences long. Having your mission statement at the top will ensure that you always keep your eyes on the target and move towards your visions on a daily basis. Make it a habit to write your top priorities along with each necessary action step every time you sit down to journal.

Step #2: Keep it simple and consistent.

Everyone's time is limited so I recommend that you keep it simple by setting a maximum of 3-5 goals or priorities related to your rehab and performance each day. Stick to your most important priorities with your journal; for example, writing about your 30-minute abdominal routine down to each set and repetition is not necessary. If core work is a priority for your performance, state the unique part of the core program for that day — perhaps you are looking to focus on a plank progression, or improving your spine alignment with a specific exercise. Focus on the bigger picture while outlining some specific details of your program which you want to keep at the top of your mind.

Step #3: Set a priority level for each goal.

Give each priority a rating broken down from most to least important. Focus on the most important goals first and make sure to plan a specific block of time during the day for each goal, if possible. If a goal doesn't get put in your calendar, then you run a higher risk of not getting it done.

Step #4: Leave space to record some general thoughts.

Leave some space and time each day to write about your mindset, level of recovery, soreness, and symptoms throughout the day. This is also a good place to record any questions you might have for your performance team. Putting these thoughts down helps as a reference, to affirm your goals, and to stay focused. Instead of overthinking certain thoughts throughout the day, writing in the journal allows you to not forget important elements without them constantly haunting you. It also lets you easily look back on your progress when you've reached a plateau and need some motivation to keep climbing.

Step #5: Include your overall effort level.

Use a 1-5 or 1-10 scale to grade your effort level, with the higher numbers indicating a maximal effort. After your workout, or near the end of the day, record this rating next to each physical task you perform for that day. This will be covered in more depth in the load management chapter.

The goal for all of the above steps is consistency and simplicity, which are also the themes of this book. Give journaling a shot and be creative with this process; try it out and see what works for you. Modify the method if you need too, that's fine. For example, writing notes on your mobile device works too, if you can maintain a specific format and keep to it on a daily basis.

To give you a sense of what a journal entry might look like. Here is an example of one from a collegiate baseball pitcher who had shoulder surgery:

Mission: Get drafted by a professional baseball team.

Daily Priorities

1. Complete Throwing Program at 1pm
   a. Action Step: Work on shoulder mobility before throwing
   b. Action Step: Complete step 5 of program for 2x20 throws at 75 feet
   c. Action Step: Take 1 minute video of my throwing & send to coach

2. Complete Post-Throwing Arm Care Routine at 2pm
   a. Complete Day 2 of Arm Care Rotator Cuff Band Routine
   b. Send video to my rehab advisor and find out if my form looks good

3. Perform Lower Body Workout at 2:30pm
   a. Complete Lower Body Mobility and Corrective Exercises
   b. Follow Workout Program: Week 3 Day 2
   c. Make sure to maintain good spine & knee alignment during squat

General Comments of the day

Morning: I woke up feeling some soreness in the back of my shoulder
Afternoon: I felt much better after warming up and was able to complete my throwing program without any issues. ***Throwing exertion felt like a 3/5**
Evening: Felt good about how today went and looking forward to increasing my throwing distance next session.

Questions: What can I do to decrease my shoulder soreness in the morning?

Get Grit

If you are sick of hearing about the mind, sit tight, we'll get to the physical side of things in the next chapter. First, it is time to talk about grit! You might be familiar with the work of psychologist Dr. Angela Duckworth, author of the best-selling book *Grit: The Power of Passion and Perseverance*. For her work with GRIT, she received the highly-regarded MacArthur "Genius" award in 2013. Grit is defined on Duckworth's website as:

> ...passion and perseverance for long-term goals. One way to think about grit is to consider what grit isn't. Grit isn't talent. Grit isn't luck. Grit isn't how intensely, for the moment, you want something. Instead, grit is about having what some researchers call an "ultimate concern"—a goal you care about so much that it organizes and gives meaning to almost everything you do. And grit is holding steadfast to that goal. Even when you fall down. Even when you screw up. Even when progress toward that goal is halting or slow.

In her preliminary research, Dr. Duckworth collaborated with some colleagues to look at factors related to success in West Point Military Academy cadet applicants and found that their grit score, a five-point scale made up of ten questions (higher score indicating higher levels of grit), was directly correlated to their success in the program. Lower dropout rates were found in cadets who had higher scores at their time of induction. Duckworth found that the grit score was actually a better measure of their ability to succeed in the program than their actual composite entrance scores which factored in their high school GPA, physical fitness score, and nominations for entrance.

Her findings have been widely applied to many high-achieving professions and elicited the same findings. This inspired her push for adoption of grit training in the education system to underprivileged students. I encourage you to go to her website[8] and take the test yourself to see your score. In just a few short minutes you will be given your grit score for free. Since I started to administer this test in my

---

[8] www.angeladuckworth.com/grit-scale

own practice, I've noticed that those with higher scores (scores of 4 and greater) tended to correlate with better coping during their rehab.

In December of 2018, I hosted a workshop called "Hacking the Off-Season For The Elite Baseball Player" at UCLA in collaboration with the cognitive-perceptual training company, Neurovision. I shared the following quote with the audience: "Grit without skill doesn't go very far, skill without grit doesn't go very far, skill coupled with grit goes very far." This quote emerged from my reflections on working with successful Major League Baseball players who seemed to have a superior work ethic along with superior skills compared to many of their minor league colleagues. One may think that players at the higher levels don't have to work as hard — that skill exonerates them from effort — but I observed the opposite. The more successful big leaguers certainly had the means to indulge in travel, the arts, and entertainment, but this was on top of their efforts. How does one get gritty so that they too can enjoy this level of success?

During an *Injured to Elite* podcast interview with John Denney, he dropped some serious knowledge on this subject when we were discussing the high performance mindset, he said: "Are you going to win to be happy, or be happy to win?" Being happy to win requires passion, which is one of the two main elements that builds grit along with perseverance according to Dr. Duckworth. John shared how some of the PGA tour golfers he coached would make statements like "I play better angry," and this is where John was able to interject with a different perspective for these individuals; passion requires loving what it is you are doing, so when you need to increase your grittiness, that is when you need to be more in tune with your passion and love of the activity you're returning to. It is much easier to persevere through challenges coming from a place of passion and love than anger.

During my undergraduate college years, when I was into my heavy lifting days as a pseudo-bodybuilder (or as my family members call it my box physique days), I came up with a method to instantaneously pump up my grit when going under a heavy load during an exercise such as a barbell bench press or heavy back squat. When I was at the gym looking around for a spotter, I would look around the area for the biggest, most muscular, individual I could find to come over and spot me during the exercise — this was a big contrast with me, a 5'6" young man on a good day height-wise. Not only was the weight almost too heavy for me to lift, but now the individual that was there to potentially save me from that heavy weight would witness firsthand my extraordinary ability to show off my strength pound-for-pound! Somehow, the idea that these big guys might doubt my abilities motivated me more than when I worked with those who knew I could do it. Plus, if I were to fail with the bigger person as a spotter, who cares? They'd be there to grab the weight.

Instead of shying away from fierce competitors, or from the more experienced individuals in your activity, rise up and surround yourself with the more skilled people. That way, you have everything to gain since there's no expectation that you'll be on-par with them! Here you are using doubt to fuel courage just as you are turning your negative Time Zero into a positive transformation. As a matter of fact, in her book *Grit*, Dr. Duckworth shares her findings that there might even be scientific evidence that we are better able to deal with adversity later in life after having experienced it at an earlier time and working through it. Going through your physical obstacle can serve as a grit-building time in your life that serves you even later in life with unrelated circumstances.

Dr. Duckworth shares the power of optimistic self-talk and a growth mindset (as opposed to a fixed mindset) about our own abilities. In my own situation, as an athlete, perhaps it was being smaller physically at a young age that gave me the room to develop a growth mindset. It is healthy to see potential in ourselves and optimism is the key; all humans have the ability to grow mentally. So grow your grit by first imagining your potential over the long-term, and second thinking about how the challenge contributes to your greater purpose. Not only will this help you persevere, but, according to Dr. Duckworth, this type of mental exercise will help grow your grit score. I always look towards what I can become and use that in moments when I find myself struggling.

Building Momentum

Before your Time Zero, you were likely less aware of your physical limitations, and probably more accustomed to going full speed when in practice and competition. After an injury, however, we tend to become hyper-aware of every thought and feeling related to our body. In the return-to-play process, some performers are so eager that they push too hard early on and quickly find their new limits. Working backwards from where they want to be is one strategy for a high performer, but can be risky as your level of physical tolerance is now much lower. On the other extreme, some performers spin their wheels and delay trying to overcome their fear of restarting their physical activities. In my experience, the best return is always gradual and progressive, gaining momentum over time instead of bouncing back and forth with the rehabilitation process.

This momentum is crucial in the Injured to Elite philosophy. Overcoming your physical adversity has the power to carry you way beyond any place you ever dreamed of taking your performance. Even seemingly negative circumstances can lead to new positive energy in your life, though it may take some time to see this full transformation. From my experience working with high-level athletes, I assure you that it is worth the wait. The key is to learn to embrace the small victories during your first few steps returning to your activity instead of hurtling forward to make a full return as soon as possible.

Gradually building momentum will safeguard you from missing critical steps in the process, and ultimately will be the quickest and safest path forward. As I mentioned in a previous chapter, cheating through the process will only end up hurting you in the long run. A common example is an athlete that returns to their activity as soon as their injured part feels back to normal without putting in the time to recondition the rest of their body. If you have ever wondered why some athletes are injury-prone, many times it is because they skip steps, only to injure another part of their body. Learning the law of momentum can help you own this part of the process, which starts in the mind.

Going a little deeper, in the book *The Tools*, authors Phil Stutz and Barry Michels talk about the higher force of forward motion, a concept very similar to momentum. When you put things slowly into action, overcoming fear and stagnation, the universe will supply you with energy you need, much like the snowball effect. Think of this in relation to your return-to-play process. If you are a skier, using this concept starts with deciding to put on a ski! It is important to break down the steps first in the mind and focus on each without forgetting the bigger picture. Skip ahead too soon, and you will mess with the law of forward motion. Now, once your skis are on then the universe supplies you with gravity which works together with the efficient movements of your body to help you slide down the mountain. However, if you miss this step by, for example, arranging your body inefficiently, then you miss the infinite supply of energy from the higher force of forward motion placing you on an optimal pathway forward. If you follow this then you will find that the gaps between where you are at currently and your ultimate vision will slowly fill in on their own. At times a little nudge in the right direction from your performance team may be all that you need.

Curing Thought Viruses

I first learned about "thought viruses" from the book *Explain Pain* by Drs. David Butler and Lorimer Moseley, and it has influenced my treatment philosophy as a performance-oriented clinician ever since. Drs. Butler and Moseley define thought viruses as a thought which indicates extreme danger in you and can be expressed through your senses as things you say, and things you think, and believe. A few practical examples of this are phrases or thoughts like "I am always going to be in pain," or "I am never going to be able to perform as well as I did before." Others, like Dr. David Coppola have defined thought viruses as "...subconscious patterns that become ingrained in our being."[9][10] In episode 12 of my *Injured to Elite* podcast "Thought

9   From Dr. Coppola's 2013 article "Thought Viruses" which can be found here: https://drdavidcoppola.com/wp-content/uploads/2016/08/Thought-Viruses.pdf
10   More details on thought viruses can be found at the *noijam* blog: https://noijam.com/2016/03/09/

Vaccines: The Cure to Thought Viruses," John Denney and I discuss how thought viruses can be positive or negative just like good and bad bacteria, both of which can spread. It is primarily negative thought viruses that slow us down or stop us entirely, so I want to introduce you to some "thought vaccines" to help you work through those negative patterns.

Self-monitor and acknowledge when you experience a negative thought virus

Whenever you catch yourself in a thought or feeling that lives in a state of fear or hopelessness, take a moment to pause and note it. You can think of it as catching yourself saying a curse word around a child. At first, they will be difficult to catch, but don't get frustrated, you are only at the beginning of rehabbing your mindset.

Below is a list of some common negative thought viruses that I have encountered with the thoughts of my clients and patients. These are examples of what you should watch out for:
- This pain isn't going away.
- Will I ever be pain-free?
- My rehab seems to be going so slow.
- This swelling seems to be here forever.
- If I can't get out of pain, I don't know how I can go on!
- Will I ever be able to play at my best again?
- This injury has ruined my life!
- How come my clinician just can't fix me?

Create and cue in your anchor switch to move forward after noting a negative thought virus.

For our purposes, an anchor switch is a self-cue that may consist of a physical movement, word, or phrase that triggers you to take control of the state that you are in mentally and physically. In order to create one, you must come up with an easily repeatable action such as a

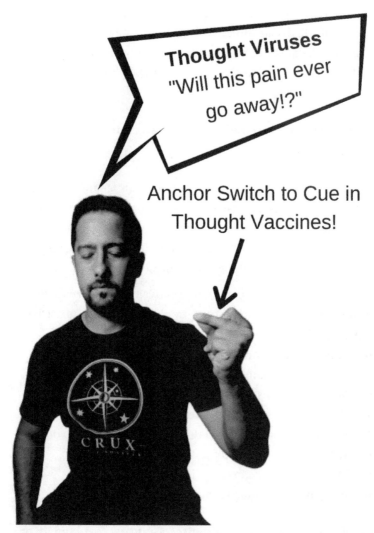

quiet snap of the finger, a self-repeated word or phrase, or even a shrug of the shoulders, something few other people will even notice. This self-created anchor will help induce a change of physiological, mental, and emotional states in order to move forward towards your goal. After you make a mental note of yourself experiencing this negative thought virus, quickly move to the next step.

You can also cue your anchor at a moment when a coach, trainer, teammate, colleague, family member, or a physical sensation is having an impact on your state of mind and body that's making it difficult for you to concentrate on your objectives. In a way, the anchor can work a bit like a secret weapon, a button only you have access to that protects you by activating your self-regulatory abilities and positive mindset.

Replace your negative thought virus with a positive thought vaccine

In an earlier section, I talked about positive affirmation statements — these are doubly important for us since they can also be used as a thought vaccine. Positive affirmation statements or "I am" statements can help us break through the negative thoughts which have the power to derail a productive day very quickly.

To move from your current state as influenced by your Time Zero to the elite place you want to be requires an affirmation of that vision. This is not about faking the thought, it's about reprogramming your way of thinking. For thought vaccines to work, your mind and body must believe them. Do you truly believe that you can affirm your visions into reality? If the answer is no, this is the area where you need to do the most rehabbing of your mind.

Once you've recognized a negative thought virus and cued your anchor, you should use a positive affirmation statement phrased "I am _____". Fill in the blank to include a statement that moves you towards your vision. Below are a few simple, yet effective, examples of these affirmations:

- ◆ I am healthy
- ◆ I am healing
- ◆ I am stronger
- ◆ I am recovering
- ◆ I am playing again
- ◆ I am performing again

As you can probably tell by now, I am a strong believer in putting in the same time and effort into developing strong mental health and a mindset of growth and resilience, as one puts into exercising the body. This belief is front and center when a high-level athlete is injured and cannot use her body as she is used to. That's the true test of a well-rounded individual, and is a cornerstone of the Injured to Elite philosophy.

To finish off this chapter, I'd like to introduce you to a tool that, like the anchor switch mentioned earlier, can be thought of as something of an invisible superpower.

Creating and Using an Alter Ego

Rich Roll is a retired lawyer who reinvented himself as a vegan ultra-endurance athlete by running in ultramarathons and other torturous events. As it happens, he also has an excellent podcast! In episode 422 of *The Rich Roll Podcast* ("Todd Herman on The Alter Ego Effect: Unlocking The Hero Within"), he featured performance expert Todd Herman who wrote a book *The Alter Ego Effect: The Power of Secret Identities To Transform Your Life.*

In that episode, Herman recounted a powerful story where, shortly before heading onstage at a conference, he ran into one of the greatest athletes of all time, Hall of Fame baseball and football player, Bo Jackson. Jackson asked him about his presentation, and Herman responded that it was about alter egos. After hearing this, Jackson turned around and said without any expression: "Bo Jackson never played a down of football." Jackson later explained that on game days, his alter ego was Jason of *Friday the 13th*. This made sense since Bo Jackson was known to be extremely aggressive on the football field. Clearly, he leveraged this alter ego to create a superhuman-like presence on the gridiron, though he was not anything like this off the field.

Think back to your own childhood, have you ever used an alter ego? Did you perhaps play pretend as a superhero like Batman or Superman? If so, how did it make you feel? When I think back to my childhood I recall home videos where I'm running around in a Batman costume telling my parents "Hey look, I'm Batman!" This type of imaginative play helps uplift and empower us to feel like we can do anything. As we grow older, however, we are told to behave and act "normal," and it becomes easy to forget that our imagination can be an extremely powerful force in our adult life, too, especially as a high performer.

Remember the topic of mirror neurons and mental imagery in relation to how we want to move or perform an activity from chapter 2? The same holds true when we want to build a persona to tap into when performing. After listening to Rich Roll's interview with Todd Herman, I started to play around with having the athletes create and tap into their own alter ego. Many of these individuals felt powerless after suffering a physical injury, so I asked them to come up with an alter ego identity that made them feel nearly invincible. I encouraged them to make up their own character if they could. Many would name professional athletes that they admired and would successfully put themselves in that frame of mind even in their injured states. This shift in persona allowed them to go from feeling demoralized to confident in their rehab process.

Steps to Building Your Alter Ego

Step #1:

Think of a fictional character or real person that embodies the character attributes and persona that you wish to possess. It can be a Hall of Fame athlete, superhero, or even a fully imagined character of your own. I recommend trying several different alter-egos to see which one works best for you.

Step #2:

Just like you created an anchor for moments when you experience a negative thought virus earlier in this chapter, you can use a similar trigger to put yourself into the shoes of your alter ego. Think of Clark Kent going into a phone booth and coming out as Superman. When you are in need of a maximum amount of grittiness immediately cue yourself into this character. You got this!

Step #3:

Refine and modify this process as needed. Don't mistake this tool as an attempt to create an arrogant identity. Many of the athletes you see on TV only appear this way because they are utilizing an identity to empower them in high-demand competitive situations. During my time working with professional athletes, I noted that many seemed like different people on and off of the field. With that in mind, I recommend you make sure to learn how to switch this alter ego off and on at appropriate times so as not to damage important relationships when not performing. Athletes who struggle to turn their alter egos off are often those that are featured in tabloid articles detailing their tumultuous relationships and addictions.

If you are interested in learning more about this tool, I highly encourage you to read the aforementioned *Alter Ego Effect: The Power of Secret Identities To Transform Your Life.*

You Made It!

Congratulations! You have now learned top strategies and tools to tap into a peak performance mindset which will take you well on your way from injured to elite. Whenever you find yourself stuck in your thoughts refer back to this chapter and review the tools and concepts presented here. Truth be told, this will all require a lot of practice, and patience, along with trial and error, just like any other part of your skills and performance. Don't gloss over this section— make a commitment to overhauling your mindset with these easily implemented tools. Even moreso, I encourage you to check out the books and websites I mentioned as my own inspirations for these topics. What I've provided here are just introductions to, for example, meditation — a topic that has been written about since ancient times.

In reviewing this chapter, we discussed pain science, thought viruses, momentum, journaling, meditation, grit, the reset breath, and the use of alter egos. These are some of the most effective tools and concepts I have integrated into the Injured to Elite method, you are the hero of your story, so don't feel like you have to limit yourself to what's outlined in this chapter; if you find other ways to improve your mindset that I haven't mentioned, then I fully encourage you to use those strategies as well. Now that you have armed your mind, it is time to connect it to the body. Taking control of your thoughts and emotions, will allow you to optimally load the rest of your body during the rehab process.

Part II: The Physical Body

"Believe me, the reward is not so great without the struggle."

–Wilma Rudolf, Sprinter

CHAPTER 6
LOAD, RECOVER, AND PROGRESS

Welcome to part two of *Injured to Elite*. This section will focus on the physical elements related to your progression. Now that you have optimized your mindset and learned how to better utilize your emotions to move towards your performance-related goals after injury, it is time to focus on optimizing your physiological state.

In this chapter, I want you to think past the conventional thought of simply "rehabbing" your injury, to training your body to adapt to increased demands while becoming more resilient. In this new world of performance optimization amongst athletes, load management and recovery have become two of the hottest terms. Let's start by talking about what recovery and load management actually mean, along with ways to help you feel in control of these concepts.

Defining Recovery

The field of sports performance requires that a multidisciplinary team strive towards common goals, but from slightly different perspectives. For example, if the team were creating a rehab program for a pitcher who just underwent elbow surgery, the strength and conditioning coordinator would be tasked with ensuring that the athlete starts a re-conditioning program, whereas the rehabilitation coordinator's top priority early on would be to protect the healing surgical area, answering to the team surgeon. As teams are putting rehab, athletic training, along with strength and conditioning under one roof, the fine line between these professions has never been more blurred.

In 2015, when I was working for the Cardinals, I had a memorable conversation with my counterpart at the time, baseball's first female professional strength and conditioning coordinator, Rachel Balkovec (now hitting coach for the New York Yankees). Rachel and I were discussing how we defined recovery as well as a potential presentation topic for one of the junior strength coaches. Since I am often drawn to looking at questions through a big-picture philosophical lens, I asked everyone in the room to give me their specific definitions of recovery. While I am unable to recall a specific answer that any of us came up with at that time, it occurred to me that defining recover, this overused word, might not be as simple as it appears to be with relation to sports performance. So then: What is recovery, and is it a state that you ever fully achieve?

Over my 15 years in the sports performance world, I have grown to believe that recovery is a process that our body undergoes when pushed to its limit for the purpose of adapting and growing into conditions both internal and external. This is the phenomenon that allows elite performers to repeatedly push themselves to their limits. Recovery is a process rather than a temporary state. In order to understand how this adaptive growth occurs, we must also understand the concept of load management. Managing load is a very active process, whereas recovery can be looked at as more of a passive physiological process that occurs naturally in the body.

Load Management

Managing your load allows you more direct ways to actively enhance your recovery, rather than trying to "hack" the recovery process. I've mentioned this before, but the human body is designed to recover from tissue damage. This feature is used in many orthopaedic surgical procedures that deliberately stimulate a healing response by moderately provoking some level of tissue damage. Some of these procedures include microfracture for cartilage damage, and tendon repair procedures which can include small drilling into bone to improve tendon-bone healing.

Stimuli that increase or decrease the load on tissue can be seen as different stressors. Think about how you manage your workload as a student or employee. When work piles up, you begin to focus on ways to lessen your mental stress by exercising or venting to a loved one, but oftentimes, in order to lessen the load, you just need to work harder to get through the pile of work. There are strategies to do that, for example, it might help to break up the hours you spend each day on given tasks. The key here is not distracting yourself or letting off steam, but managing the actual stressor.

This directly relates back to your performance-related goals; while there are many flashy new recovery tools on the market, they are often much less powerful than using intelligent strategies to manage your overall workload. The amazing thing about the human body is its ability to adapt to the demands we ask of it. Ask too much, and you risk exceeding tissue tolerance, ask too little and you'll see little to no improvement. After Time Zero, some pushing is necessary or else your body will take the path of least resistance and you will remain at zero. The way towards elite performance is to use momentum to drive progress.

Before I say anything else, I want you to know that the two most important elements to recovery are nutrition and sleep; humans were tired and hungry long before any gym, therapist, or cryotherapy device existed. To put it bluntly: Our recovery is heavily influenced by what we eat and the quality of our sleep. That's why sleep and nutrition will be covered later in this chapter. For now, I want to focus on progressing load after injury.

Don't Stop Moving

In the early years of medicine, people were often told to simply rest after injury. Back in the early-20th century, people were put in body casts after breaking bones, bed rest was the answer to lower back

pain, and even in more recent times, we instructed our patients to keep
their leg elevated with an ice pack after an ankle sprain. Fast-forward
to the 21st century and people are dealing with higher rates of chronic
back pain. A 2008 study called "The Rising Prevalence of Chronic Low
Back Pain"[11] found a significant increase in the prevalence of lower
back pain from 3.9% in 1992 to 10% in 2006 among over 5,000 North
Carolina residents. This begs the question: Are we simply not as "gritty"
as our ancestors? Has an older family member ever told you how times
were just harder for them when they were growing up? We've all heard
the joke about how in the olden times, they had to walk to school
in the snow, uphill both ways. Perhaps with the advent of modern
rehabilitation in the 20th century, fear of further injury led to a culture
of pushing the panic button after even the smallest of injuries. We can
only wonder if this has brought us to higher rates of disability from
common conditions like back pain.

In the world of rehabilitation, the tide has recently shifted to
where we now realize it can be more harmful than helpful to fully step
off the gas pedal after an injury. Instead, we now recommend early
"mobilization" after injury. As I tell clients, don't misinterpret this as
an endorsement to run through walls, rather it's a request that you ask
a bit more of your body than you might feel like right after injury. For
instance, taking a day off from the field after a low-grade ankle sprain
is expected, but staying in bed for several days can inhibit your ability
to go from injured to elite. In chapter five, I mentioned that negative
thoughts can spread like viruses. Indeed, the messages we send our
body, whether we encourage movement or avoid it, can determine the
level of momentum that is built up in every stage of the process; objects
in motion stay in motion, said Isaac Newton. They say he was a smart
guy!

When beginning the rehabilitation process with a patient who
has a significant limitation in range of motion, I use the phrase "motion
is lotion" to encourage them to move early on. Managing load right
after injury requires the ability to tap into the "Goldilocks Principle."

---

11   Freburger, J. K., Holmes, G. M., Agans, R. P., Jackman, A. M., Darter, J. D., Wallace, A. S., Castel, L. D., Kalsbeek, W. D., & Carey, T. S. (2009). The rising prevalence of chronic low back pain. *Archives of internal medicine*, 169(3), 251-258. https://doi.org/10.1001/archinternmed.2008.543

Those who recall the story of Goldilocks remember hearing about the porridge that was just right. In the same way, your goal is to find what amount of load and movement is *just right* for you and your injury. Below are the steps to managing your own load and recovery:

Step #1: Follow the goldilocks "just right" principle of progression. Meet in the middle of the two extreme ideas of don't do anything in pain and "no pain no game." [12]

Striving to perform the optimal amount of work without over or under doing it is certainly not simple, but there are a few concepts which can make it easier to identify a balance on your own. As we discussed in previous chapters, after an injury, the tissue in that area may be more vulnerable so your body utilizes pain as an early warning system. This is one way the sympathetic (fight or flight) nervous system along with the limbic system (primitive area of your brain) work to thwart threats. Keep in mind that the brain and body aren't always right about a perceived threat (remember the earlier example of the over-sensitive AI on new cars?). While oftentimes threats are not nearly as dangerous as your system interprets, if we ignore our mind and body's reactions, they often respond more strongly — just like a car might automatically brake even if there is plenty of distance between you and another object. Systems like these are designed for maximum self-preservation, not elite performance and so they tend to err on the side of caution.

For this reason, we want to incrementally increase our baseline level of activity without over-activating the body's alert systems. In order to do that, you can think of your activity progression as a mission to stay under the radar. While they may be unpleasant, discomfort and soreness can be good indicators that your tissue is responding to the

---

12   With regards to those professionals who say: "If it hurts, don't do it!" I want to point out a possible unintended negative psychological effect. If we condition ourselves to look for the pain, guess what we will be intuitively more likely to find? Pain! In contrast, it is wise to look for what you would rather feel, such as smooth fluid motion, as you will be in a more receptive psychological state to find just that. When we are faced with the intense feelings of pain during our ascent, it can be very freeing to simply be present with it and allow it to just do its thing. This is a true state of being present with yourself. Not trying to do much of anything. Mastering this is a key to moving fluidly through your action plan from Injured to Elite.

load. A moderate amount of load is fine, so don't fall into the trap of thinking that you must shut down if you begin to feel some unpleasant sensations.

Keeping to this "just right" principle is where the art of being a rehabilitation expert comes into play. Some clinicians (especially the more conservative physical therapists) instruct their patient to watch out for pain — that it should never accompany an exercise or activity. On the other extreme, there are clinicians out there who use phrases like "no pain, no game" to empower their patients. Going to either extreme can be dangerous in the long run, and the reason why someone with my skillset was in a job managing the rehabilitation process for professional baseball players; if I didn't push them at all they would never go back to playing, and if I pushed them too hard, I might push them out of the game. So I had to use a combination of my book knowledge and powers of observation to find just the right approach to keep the rehabilitation process flowing smoothly.

In my job as a Rehab Coordinator, I was often put on the spot by the higher-ups in the front office who were in charge of baseball operations and player transactions — they'd want to know a specific timeline for when players would be ready to play at full capacity. I could only be right some of that time, as normally the player would either be ready a bit sooner or a bit later than expected. This is one of the parts of being a Rehab Coordinator I didn't enjoy; it felt wrong for the team and I to decide what we thought was most appropriate instead of allowing the process to be fully owned by the player. That experience is a major reason why a cornerstone of the Injured to Elite method is empowering you to take full ownership of your recovery and worry less about answering to others. If you stay focused on the next step with an understanding of your own journey, then you need not worry exactly when it will happen. Rather, you can spend your energy exploring the how.

Pushing the athlete adequately required a logical and incremental progression where they were an active participant. The more on-board an athlete was with the plan, meaning the more steps of the plan they participated in creating, the better the outcome.

This is part of the reason I'm teaching you how to become your own rehabilitation expert; the more involved you are, the higher the chances you'll leave the injury behind and be stronger than ever before. Keeping the philosophy of incremental progress while staying just under the body's radar (and the pain that accompanies it), yet still pushing your activities forward is key. In the next few steps you will learn how to understand your level of exertion in order to determine the right intensity to keep moving forward without disrupting your optimal recovery path. Before that though, you need to determine what your specific destination will be, and set that intention.

Step #2: In order to manage your load and recovery, you must first know your destination and then reverse-engineer the pathway.

What is the first thing you do when you're not sure how to get somewhere? That's right, you type the destination address into your GPS. Once you know your destination and goal, it is much easier to reverse-engineer your path. In our case, what is your recovery goal, and what are the steps on the route to get there? These steps will serve as the many landmarks along your route. I would say that my top skill as a performance coach and physical therapist is figuring out the steps to recovery that might not be as visible to the naked eye. For example, with a baseball pitcher, if the goal is to fully return to pitching, what amount of throwing is needed before starting back on the mound, and what does the athlete need to do to get to that point?

The truth is that there could be an almost-infinite number of steps and variables along that progression. The trick is to understand the priorities and figure out the simplest steps between them. I advise you to put in as many steps in-between your destination and where you currently are as possible. Use these steps to guide your actions when you hit a roadblock. At that moment, you might want to go over the last successful step and repeat as necessary. If needed, go back a step further, and once that step is completed successfully again, move ahead. If there is doubt or concern, or a lack of confidence, repeat the step. Once you are satisfied with it, move on. Always ask yourself, what really makes sense next? Is there a smaller step that I might be missing? Luckily, we can all fall back on the ability to figure this out through trial and error. When we push the gas too hard, our innate systems give us feedback including a general sense of energy reserve. What is your energy reserve monitor to go from injured to elite?

Step #3: Driving up the mountain after injury requires energy and momentum.

Think of energy as load, and momentum as recovery. This occurred to me as Olya and I were driving on I-70 through the state of Colorado. The road was never fully uphill, rather it was bouts of altitude increases followed by drops over and over again. I noticed an interesting phenomenon when making this drive: Whenever completing yet another bout of going uphill, peaking, and going downhill once more, over time we still ended up gaining altitude. It was almost as if the altitude drop after each climb gave us the momentum to make our slow and steady climb. Another example is a bobsled flying down an Olympic track, picking up tremendous speed by making massive altitude drops and then shooting right back up around steep twists and turns.

In many ways, a journey through an injury follows this path; you put in the work going uphill, but then allow the body to undergo intermittent states of much-needed recovery, and get at it again keeping that momentum going forward back uphill. If you fully let go of the gas pedal, you will eventually stop, and if you don't step off the gas pedal you will either veer off the road or run out of gas; your time after injury is unlikely to be a fully linear journey towards peak performance. Because of this fact, you must learn how to harness your energy while not over-exerting yourself before your tissue has time to build up resilience. When your body is talking to you in pain, this is your primitive nervous system saying: "Are you sure that you want to be doing this to me after we just got injured?" During the time after an injury, we need to gradually teach this older, more primitive, part of the brain that it is okay and, in fact, necessary to build resilience. Naturally, this involves some pain.

So the question is, if we use this analogy of driving through the Rocky Mountains, how does one know how high to drive before going back down slightly and then trekking on? On a driving trip, you have the road to tell you, but how about with an injury? The answer is an intuitive one, you've got to figure out your destination first! When I drove through the Rocky Mountains, I knew the path to follow that would lead me to Denver. Had I not known my destination, I couldn't have possibly known how much gas was needed nor how to manage that energy wisely, much less what exit to take. So to bring it back to the injury, creating your progression requires that you know both your destination and how to measure your energy level.

Knowing your destination is fairly straightforward, though it's different for everyone. If your destination is to run a marathon and you are training like a football player, it might be time to reconsider your approach. Generally, though, your destination can be a specific movement you want to achieve, or more widely, a full and most pain-free return to your sport (which is a combination of specific movements). In considering this, ask yourself whether your goal is simply to return to your pre-injury self, or is it to get on the trajectory to surpass your previous capabilities? This is the question that should be echoing in your mind as you work with your team to determine your progression.

Once you've thought about it and defined your destination, it is time to build your own performance energy gauge and altimeter to know the correct amount of exertion needed to be used for specific tasks.

Step #4: Monitor your energy reserve in order to get you to the destination.

There are a few ways to easily monitor your exertion and fatigue level. The old school method, which has been heavily researched, is called the rate of perceived exertion (RPE). The new school method, on the other hand, looks at your heart rate variability as an indicator that many believe will show your overall level of "recovery." RPE in its simplest form, is a scale from 1 to 10 with a 1 indicating very light exertional activity to a 10 indicating maximal effort. Each can correlate to a certain percentage of your maximum heart rate and specific training zones, however we don't need to get that technical here.

When I write out arm care programs for professional baseball players, I incorporate an even simpler three-point fatigue scale. I ask the athlete to rate their level of fatigue for each day of the program with a one being minimal fatigue, two being moderate fatigue, and three being a state of maximum fatigue. The more fatigue, the less gas you have, and the more immediate recovery you require. While this scale can certainly be criticized, the Injured to Elite process seeks simplicity where possible, allowing you to attend to the more important things. I have found that the more complex you make this effort/fatigue grading system the more confusing your process forward will feel; nobody likes when every light pops up on your dashboard and it becomes impossible to figure out what's going on. In that situation, you won't be going anywhere other than to your mechanic, or in this case, right to your clinician.

The goal here is not to keep your fatigue level at a constant one, since like leaving your foot off the gas, you will get nowhere. Rather, you should use your fatigue level to determine your priority for the day. Make sure that your journal entries include a space for your RPE, and feel free to use that space to record not only your overall fatigue level, but also a specific step or activity you completed for the day. If an activity was rated at a one out of three (3-point scale) for several sessions in a row, then it might be time to progress to the next logical step towards your physical goal by adding load. If you rate an activity or your overall fatigue at a 3/3, don't increase past your current step until it gets to a two or lower.

Another scale I use is one that helps determine how difficult an exercise or activity should be, or to answer the question: How many sets and reps should I perform? It's a 5-point activity effort scale with the following points (see illustration on next page):

**INJURED TO ELITE 1-5 EFFORT SCALE
TO GRADE ACTIVITY INTENSITY**

1	MINIMAL EFFORT: BASELINE ACTIVITY LEVEL
2	LEARNING OR RE-LEARNING A NEW MOVEMENT/SKILL
3	PERFORMING A REHAB OR CORRECTIVE EXERCISE
4	TRAINING AND LOADING A BODY PART
5	MAX EFFORT: PERFORMANCE ENHANCEMENT

1. Baseline Activity
2. Learning or Re-Learning a New Movement/Skill
3. Performing a Rehab or Corrective Exercise
4. Training and Loading the Body or Body Part
5. Performance Enhancement

Thinking of all exercises, movements, and activities you do on this 5-point scale can help you determine how much volume of a specific task you should be performing by determining if the intensity level of effort (on the previous RPE scale) matches the activity on this 5-point scale. If the activity does not match the effort level, then you can manipulate the amount of sets, repetitions, duration, or load to keep yourself on track.

Follow along with this example to better understand the use of this scale to effectively apply it to your training. If an American football player's goal is to increase their 40-yard dash time while they are completing a sprinting session, and on the 5-point effort scale they rate it at a 3/5, as a performance enhancement activity, they are lacking effort. The athlete should increase their effort to a maximum 5/5 in order to work on this intended goal as seen in the scale. However, if they are performing a rehab exercise for their recovering knee and their effort level is a 5/5 then the intensity is far too high, and they should lower their effort by decreasing the sets, reps, or load.

The biggest issue with performance enhancement, which will also be discussed in the Performance Optimization chapter, is the increased risk of injury as we increase our intensity to maximal efforts. This is not to suggest you should not get to maximum levels, but that you make sure you do your best job of self-monitoring when you are at the top of your effort levels. Just like most cars have speed governors which limit their top speed to prevent a breakdown, spikes in absolute peak performance levels are the most dangerous points when striving for elite performance, especially after injury. If you're planning to go all out, do it wisely and under the guidance of your team members. Returning to my previous point about defining your destination, if you know the path, as long as you plan for these peak effort moments at certain points in your journey, it will be easy to also plan post-peak performance recovery sessions.

Let's return quickly to the section about utilizing momentum. When you're training for recovery, keeping traction is key — we know that slamming on the gas always comes with a price. Breaking momentum can result in spinning your wheels when attempting to push too hard. So keep going, growing and recovering day by day. Rest assured that even if you don't see your "numbers" going up, you are still likely benefitting in other areas of your life. Think about it, you are a person in control. You have a team on your side and a plan to surpass your best former self. And even when you're struggling, you are demonstrating and building up your grit by overcoming physical and mental challenges. Every day, you are becoming the person you want to be as you go from injured to elite!

Fancier Modern Ways of Measuring Your Own Recovery

Some of the latest advances in technology related to recovery monitoring and optimization utilize a concept called heart rate variability. Heart rate variability measures the time interval in-between heartbeats known as the "RR interval" on an electrocardiogram. One heartbeat cycle is made up of electrical activity known as a PQRST wave and this interval looks at the change in heartbeats in milliseconds. Heart rate variability has been found in research to serve as an indicator of overall sympathetic or parasympathetic activity. Basically the lower our heart rate variability is, the more stressed and fatigued we tend to be, and the higher our heart rate variability, the more calm and composed we are. When our heart rate variability is high, that can indicate that our autonomic nervous system is very responsive at speeding up and normalizing.

Devices such as the Morpheus watch and WHOOP band are a few examples of products you can easily purchase to monitor your heart rate variability. You will want to see an overall level of recovery as well as much more in-depth data in order to determine the appropriate level of activity and training intensity to undertake. Since these devices are still new on the market, I recommend not fully relying on them. Instead, if you're interested, I suggest playing around with one and seeing if you can spot patterns that may be meaningful to your recovery process. It doesn't hurt to have more data points, after all.

The majority of the rest of this chapter is going to focus on what I, along with many others, believe to be the most important elements to optimize recovery. Although recovery is one of our body's natural abilities, disturbances in our sleep and nutrition can significantly impact our ability to optimally recover and grow. The process of both digestion and sleep occur best in a parasympathetic state, nearly always associated with a state of relaxation.

Optimizing Recovery Through Sleep

Why is sleep so important to go from injured to elite? After injury our body is already in a state of special need due to the ongoing natural healing and rebuilding process that starts right after Time Zero. This early tissue healing is an important part of the inflammatory process. I have noticed that patients tend to need more sleep after going back to their daily routine following orthopedic-related surgery.

"Further, a study published in the *Journal of Pediatric Orthopaedics* found that middle school and high school adolescent athletes in a large metropolitan area who got nine hours of sleep per night showed the lowest likelihood of injuries."[13] Sleep is the ultimate parasympathetic state for our brain and body. As a matter of fact, there are even specific brain waves called delta waves, which are the slowest waves, associated with the deep level of sleep. Short-change your sleep and you take away one of your most important allies when it comes to recovery.

If you are someone who reads about the latest and greatest in the world of high performance, then the importance of sleep is not foreign information to you. Back when I was with the Cardinals, this area of study was just heating up. At the time, we were looking at better ways to track sleep patterns and improve the quality sleep for our baseball players. After that, I have been fortunate enough to learn about sleep from Dr. William Hart, a top sleep expert in the state of California. Dr. Hart explained that there are two important aspects of sleep: Getting to sleep and staying asleep. In each of these phases, there are specific prerequisites and physiological requirements that the body must undergo. A few of the most important factors which can influence your ability to fall asleep include body temperature, thoughts, eating habits, light, and your exercise schedule. The key physiological occurrence that needs to happen prior to sleep is a decrease in core body temperature. Here are some other tips for falling asleep:

◆ Avoid working out close to your scheduled sleep time.
◆ Avoid taking a hot shower right before sleep
  ○ Try a lukewarm or cool bath or shower 1-2 hours prior to bed allowing the body enough time to cool down.
◆ Create a cool, yet comfortable, sleeping environment.
◆ Decrease the amount of blue light being emitted from your mobile device, blue light can disrupt brain waves necessary for deep sleep.
  ○ Many mobile phones these days have a built-in app that lets you schedule a decrease in blue light depending on a

13   Milewski MD, Skaggs DL, Bishop GA, et al. (2014). Chronic lack of sleep is associated with increased sports injuries in adolescent athletes. J Pediatr Orthop. 34(2):129-133. doi:10.1097/BPO.0000000000000151

preset bedtime. This is especially useful if you have kids that need a good night's sleep before school.

◆ Thoughts, anxiety, and your overall emotional state can directly impact your ability to fall asleep so find an unwinding technique that works for you. Many people read a book (as long as it's not full of suspense that'll keep you reading all night), though you can also take those few minutes to write in your performance journal.

◆ Maintain a dark room. If you're having trouble falling asleep, blackout curtains can make all of the difference, though complete darkness may take some getting used to.

◆ If you find yourself in a bit more mental unease, double up on your meditation. Many meditation apps have guided meditations specifically designed to help with sleep, but a simple body scan can also work wonders.

Once you're peacefully asleep, next up is staying asleep: If you are having issues staying asleep it is possible that there might be a physical reason related to your breathing. The most common physical reason is an obstruction of your airways, also known as sleep apnea. Since the body is designed to keep you alive at all times (even throughout the night!), a moment of disruption in your airway is enough for it to kick into action and wake you up to maintain safe breathing. Interestingly, I learned from Dr. Hart that some sleep physicians even go so far to believe that snoring is indicative of dysfunctional sleep patterns since it is related to airway obstruction.

Some risk factors for sleep apnea are neck size, being male, and excess weight. Think about how these risk factors might relate to people after injury. For example, someone who gains weight after injury due to inactivity may be at an increased risk for sleep apnea, which can then impede their performance. If you're concerned that you might be suffering from sleep apnea, there is a simple and credible questionnaire you can fill out online[14] to find out if you are at an increased risk. If you

---

14   The STOP-Bang website was put up by a research team at the University of Toronto: http://www.stopbang.ca/osa/screening.php

are concerned, I recommend that you consult with your primary care physician. And don't worry, even if you have sleep apnea, there are treatments available.

The last important concept with regards to sleep is that you can indeed change your natural circadian rhythm. Our circadian rhythm is basically our internal clock. A concept in the sports performance world is putting athletes on similar sleep schedules to allow them to sync up better during competition. During your post-injury transformation you will find that your schedule has likely changed. It is important to maintain structure to allow you to perform when you need to be at your best. If you are sleeping in till noon every day and exercising right after you wake up, or later in the afternoon, remember that you are running the risk of throwing off your circadian rhythm and internal clock for the future. Prioritize your schedule and sleep at optimal times to allow for structure in your days after injury even if you are out of work, school, or competition.

Don't get thrown off because you have some extra time on your hands, be proactive with your schedule. As a matter of fact, that extra time should be something for which you are grateful. Devote it to other passion projects or self-development areas that you weren't able to get to prior to the injury. Think about what part of the day is the most vital time for you to be at your fullest level of energy and alertness? Base your sleep schedule around this time so you could put first things first. At the same time, make sure that you keep in mind that your current schedule may very well need to change in the not-so-distant future when you are back to higher levels of activity and competition. Give yourself ample time to get back to that set schedule and train yourself to be on the right schedule well before it comes.

Remember that earlier study which found that getting more sleep lowers the risk of injury. If you ask a Navy SEAL or some high-performance gurus, they might say that we overestimate our needs. In general this might be true, but few would argue that the body's needs are higher after an injury. Use any extra time you have in your schedule to optimize your recovery, rather than potentially harm it. That means get enough sleep!

Optimizing Recovery Through Nutrition

In addition to sleep, what you eat will be one of the most important elements to optimize your recovery. Since the world certainly doesn't need another diet book, I want to keep this short. I have some strong opinions on this topic, however, you should remain an open-minded skeptic; don't let me dissuade you from your current diet if you are getting good results. Recall when we discussed the three elements of evidence-based medicine in the first section, what the research says, the experience of the clinician, and the experience of you, the individual. This is why I often repeat that if you try something, objectively measure the results, and find that it works for you, treat that as meaningful no matter what anyone else says. Go ahead and try out different diets in order to figure out what works best for your body, but make sure to follow it within reason and give yourself adequate time to assess. Recently, there has been a substantial increase in athletes attempting a vegetarian or vegan diet. That last sentence would have been looked at as crazy thirty years ago, but athletes have tried vegan diets and found that it works for them.

So why is diet and nutrition so important in relation to your recovery? Pushing the limits of your body after an injury is a process of stimulating the breakdown of both your injured and non-injured tissue. We call this a catabolic physiological process. The process by which we rebuild, recover, and grow is known as an anabolic process. Eating is essentially adding the clay to your sculpture while exercising and performing sculpts the excess clay to unleash the potential beneath. Our biology looks to maintain a state of regularity or "homeostasis" so that anabolism and catabolism happen seamlessly day in and day out, that's why one training session or one meal won't make a big difference in the long run. It is the habits you developed before and continue after your injury that will most certainly influence your long-term results.

Though I want you to do what works for you, I do have a couple of dietary suggestions specifically for when recovering from an injury. The first is that I strongly advise against "zero" carbohydrate diets, especially immediately after your Time Zero event. The reason for this is based on a very basic rule of our physiology: We use carbohydrates as our fundamental source of energy throughout the day, especially when needed quickly. Through a process called glycolysis, our body breaks down glucose. During glycogenolysis, our body breaks down our storage of glucose (glycogen) that is stored in our skeletal muscle and liver. Ensuring adequate quality complex carbohydrate intake will allow for optimal levels of glycogen stores to be replenished during intense bouts of training and recovery. Complex carbohydrates differ from simple carbohydrates in their ability to provide longer lasting energy, however they are also broken down at a slower rate. If your car operates mainly on a certain type of fuel, you would use that fuel, wouldn't you? Do the same for your body — feed it energy with quality carbohydrates! A few examples of complex carbohydrates include sweet potatoes, whole grains, and beans.

Second, I caution you from following an intermittent fasting diet during the early post-injury process. The main reason being that it doesn't factor in the varying physical demands throughout your day; it's pretty difficult to perform at a high level if you haven't eaten for hours prior. With any diet, put your priorities first and the rest shall fall into place. Avoid putting your goals into the framework of other aspects of your life. If you are truly making the commitment to go from injured to elite in your life, you need to prioritize your goals (alongside family) first. This will make decisions a lot easier throughout the day when determining your schedule, and your diet.

There is no better time in your life than after injury to make the changes you already know are best for you. Getting rid of processed foods, limiting extra sugar, and keeping to a diet high in whole foods, fruits, and vegetables will only help give your engine the premium fuel it deserves. Keep your diet simple and consistent, and you will reap the benefits of an unwavering recovery. Additionally, your nervous system will thank you ten-fold for feeding it from a good source of energy. Our brain cells, known as neurons, require healthy fats known as omega-3 fatty acids which are highly concentrated in foods such as fish and flax seeds. Keeping the brain well-fed and hydrated will set the stage for maintaining an optimized mindset. The positive feedback from an improved state of your mind will only help the rest of your journey.

Inflammation and "The Cold Hard Facts on Ice"[15]

Various forms of cryotherapy (including ice) have been some of the most widely used recovery techniques over the past several decades. Ice baths, ice massages, cold packs, ice packs, cryotherapy chambers, and cold compression therapy, are just a few of the ways people use ice after an injury. Interestingly, and contrary to widely-held beliefs in sports medicine, research is inconclusive on the effectiveness of ice for recovery and healing. This section is not intended to be a debate about heat versus ice, rather it will serve as a bit of a myth-buster regarding the prominence of icing as a recovery method.

I was encouraged to use ice early in my career and this became a very regular part of my patient's treatment. If you were a patient of mine, at the end of a session there was a good chance that you would have received some form of cryotherapy, and if you were to ask for ice I would rarely challenge the request. Once I started my work in professional baseball, ice wraps were like giving out lollipops at the barbershop. After a pitcher would come off the field, ice was a regular part of their initial recovery. But things have changed quickly in the last 5-10 years as many practitioners began to challenge more conventional thinking on this topic. It was around the time of that change that I met with Gary Reinl, a man known widely in the professional and collegiate sports world (especially in the baseball circles) as the self-proclaimed "Anti-Ice Man." In talking to him, I was impressed by his ability to break down the science of inflammation, making a strong argument against the use of ice.

Sure, Gary is part-salesman, but don't roll your eyes too quickly! He is also a well-regarded expert in the field of sports performance. In

15   Piana LE, Garvey KD, Burns H, Matzkin EG. *The Cold, Hard Facts of Cryotherapy in Orthopedics.* Am J Orthop (Belle Mead NJ). 2018;47(9):10.12788/ajo.2018.0075. doi:10.12788/ajo.2018.0075

his book, *ICED! The Illusionary Treatment Option*, Gary explains that the icing method began in the 1970s after the first successful surgical reattachment of a severed arm was stored on ice. The ice helped prevent tissue decay just like in the preservation of meat, and after this success, a leap was made that you should ice injured parts of your body, even though research on the efficacy of this remains inconclusive to this day.

To understand this scientifically, here is a general breakdown on inflammation. The inflammatory process occurs after any type of tissue injury. Although there is a strong negative connotation with the inflammatory process, any qualified medical professional will tell you that the inflammatory process is actually also a very necessary part of healing; this process is our immune system's way of attacking a threat and at the same time calling all "troops" (cells) to an area of the body in order to clean up a mess and protect from further injury. Just like any construction site produces garbage, our body produces a large amount of debris and waste products through this process of inflammation. If these waste products are not evacuated out of the area, then you are left with what we know as swelling or edema. This swelling can become problematic for a joint's range of motion, and decrease strength by inhibiting nerve impulses to muscles, as well as increasing levels of pain due to the compressed nature of the area. Anyone that has had surgery especially in the lower extremity can attest to the negative effects of swelling.

It is no surprise, then, that we are obsessed with ways to get rid of swelling in the performance world. What Gary makes self-evident however, is that it doesn't make sense to use ice to get rid of this congestion. The more recent and conventional wisdom of ice preaches that ice will serve as a vasoconstrictor, decreasing blood flow as it is believed that the cold induces certain chemical substances (neurotransmitters) such as norepinephrine to vasoconstrict blood vessels, decreasing local circulation. Decreasing blood flow to an area of swelling is thought to decrease the amount of additional swelling. However, that initial increase in circulation following the inflammatory process also includes many benefits, such as bringing those aforementioned "troops" (cells) to fight infection and patch the area up. This part of the process is exactly where the benefits of ice become confusing.

The analogy to think of is a busy highway during a rush-hour commute. Imagine having the ability to control the flow through this highway and literally freezing the traffic. What would happen if you decided to slow this traffic down even more? The exits off of the highway and the highway itself would become nothing short of a traffic jam. During Thanksgiving Day when making the commute around the tri-state metro area, the last thing anyone wants is to slow that traffic down any further. The best thing that could happen is speeding up the areas of traffic congestion which would eventually open the whole network of roads back up. The same holds true for our own body — if we slow down or freeze an area of swelling all that will happen is the circulation is delayed and the waste products stay in the area. Some even believe a rebound effect might occur which can increase the swelling in that area after using ice. For these reasons, the science behind the use of ice for swelling in many ways is counterproductive.

Even so, there are times when ice can be beneficial for recovery. For example, it does very well at numbing an area, which is useful prior to treatment for an athlete who is in extreme pain. Also, some patients are so set on receiving ice, that it provides almost a placebo effect; in those cases I'll discuss my views on the topic but certainly not withhold it since applying ice after an injury is unlikely to hurt recovery. Again, the experience of the patient or athlete does provide some evidence for practice.

Getting back to inflammation, I want to tell you how our body processes that swelling. In fact; our complex and well-designed physiology has a specific system just for this, known as the lymphatic system. This is basically a plumbing system of vessels throughout our body that filters out many waste products. There is a vast network of vessels that carry "lymph" or waste products through it with the help of another important system that I'm sure you're well aware of: The musculoskeletal system. Your voluntary and involuntary muscle contractions and movement actually stimulate the flow of the lymphatic system by pushing the waste products through the deep and more superficial traversing vessels throughout your entire body. In the world of sports performance, we utilize this innate process to enhance the idea of active recovery.

Moving on, there are a few other topics related to inflammation that are important to discuss. The use of non-steroidal anti-inflammatory medications, also known as NSAIDS, have gotten a lot of heat over the past several years. These medications that come in many forms, both prescribed and over-the-counter, basically intend to disrupt the process of inflammation. Proponents of avoiding these, feel that anti-inflammatories may inhibit initial healing and might actually have negative health-related consequences such as a recent finding in a study, which showed decreased levels of the hormone testosterone[16].

My intention is not for you to go against any medical advice you are already receiving but rather to encourage you to truly understand some of the over-the-counter pills you may be putting into your body. Many athletes have the habit of popping ibuprofen like candy, and although I am not making the statement that you should never use NSAIDs, I am against blindly taking large amounts of them, as it can possibly hinder performance. Furthermore, since these substances need to be processed by many bodily systems, including our kidneys and liver, there is a chance that the strain they put on the body will eventually catch up with you. Here are just a few of the potential hazards of overdoing NSAIDS: Gastro-intestinal distress, gastric ulcers, decreased testosterone production, and negative effects on the kidneys. As always, check with your treating physician if you have any further questions about medications.

The last point to be made in this section is the overall idea is not exactly about whether inflammation is good or bad, or if we should even focus on limiting this process. Looking at the bigger picture, our body maintains a delicate balance that sustains life through countless routine processes, including inflammation. During high levels of training and

16   Kristensen, D. M., Desdoits-Lethimonier, C., Mackey, A. L., Dalgaard, M. D., De Masi, F., Munkbøl, C. H., Styrishave, B., Antignac, J. P., Le Bizec, B., Platel, C., Hay-Schmidt, A., Jensen, T. K., Lesné, L., Mazaud-Guittot, S., Kristiansen, K., Brunak, S., Kjaer, M., Juul, A., & Jégou, B. (2018). Ibuprofen alters human testicular physiology to produce a state of compensated hypogonadism. *Proceedings of the National Academy of Sciences of the United States of America*, 115(4), E715–E724. https://doi.org/10.1073/pnas.1715035115

recovery from injury, there will almost certainly be a higher level of inflammation. Curtailing some of the negative effects of this process for more effective training, or even comfort, is certainly reasonable, but as with many things in life, moderation is key.

An Unusual Recommendation (That Works!)

Finally, I will share with you my one supplemental diet recommendation with regards to performance nutrition. There are a plethora of studies showing the benefits of tart cherry juice for recovery. To give two examples: Howatson et al (2012)[17] found that consumption of tart cherry juice by study participants increased sleep quality and duration during the trial. Likewise, findings by Levers et al (2016)[18] showed reduced immune and inflammatory stress in endurance runners and triathletes after consumption of tart cherry supplements. I first learned about the benefits of tart cherry juice early in my career as a physical therapist while sitting in on the "weekly fellow's conference" at the Nicholas Institute of Sports Medicine and Athletic Trauma. During this meeting, the topic of tart cherry juice was mentioned along with some research findings of its benefits as a natural anti-inflammatory.

Keep in mind that sports medicine research studies are careful with their claims — in that vein, it is important to mention that studies (especially as it pertains to tart cherries) usually find one must consume a high concentration of cherries to produce a statistically significant result when correlated with a bodily process or performance outcome. It isn't simply that drinking a glass of tart cherry juice will cure your tendinitis. Supplements such as tart cherry juice, and others such as essential oils offer many benefits, but as always it is only a part of a holistic healing process.

---

17   Howatson, G., Bell, P. G., Tallent, J., Middleton, B., McHugh, M. P., & Ellis, J. (2012). Effect of tart cherry juice (Prunus cerasus) on melatonin levels and enhanced sleep quality. *European journal of nutrition*, 51(8), 909-916. https://doi.org/10.1007/s00394-011-0263-7

18   Levers, K., Dalton, R., Galvan, E. et al. (2016) Effects of powdered Montmorency tart cherry supplementation on acute endurance exercise performance in aerobically trained individuals. *J Int Soc Sports Nutr* 13, 22. https://doi.org/10.1186/s12970-016-0133-z

When it comes to tart cherry juice, my advice is to get the benefit by eating organic tart cherries as one of your main snacks, just as long as you have no medical condition that would make this dangerous for you. When I worked for the Cardinals, this was a suggestion I often shared with my baseball players, and they anecdotally reported positive outcomes. Placebo? Maybe, but there is certainly research to support why some of the players I worked with continued to take this seriously. Any safe and legal edge in the world of professional baseball is of extreme value!

Beyond tart cherries, I encourage you to go out there and do your own research, experiment with sensible options, and make notes in your performance journal about how different foods and sleeping patterns affect you over time. Just don't let any snake oil salesman sell you on some crazy idea about a magic food or pill. My years as a medical professional have taught me that, while there are supplements and strategies that do make some difference in recovery, anyone making outlandish claims is probably embellishing. It's like the science fiction author, Robert Heinlein used to say: TINSTAAFL, or, there is no such thing as a free lunch; if something sounds too good to be true, it might just be.

Finally, if diet is a priority area for you then you might consider establishing a relationship with an expert, either someone on your team or an outside consultant you meet with periodically. As long as their experience and knowledge meet a high standard, let them help you eat better. Now, go grab some tart cherries before we get into a chapter about something many people have asked me about over the years: Performance optimization.

CHAPTER 7
PERFORMANCE
OPTIMIZATION

Welcome! I'm so glad you're here. You've learned about getting your mind right, the basics of sleep and nutrition, and a whole lot more. In this chapter, you're going to get the seven tools of performance that the Injured to Elite method enhances and optimizes so that you can achieve your physical goals. We'll go over more science behind some concepts that have already been mentioned, but not in a complicated or confusing way. However, if you do find yourself getting a little intimidated, just focus on the major take-home points that you can readily integrate into your program, you can always return to study the scientific explanations later. The seven tools are recovery, athleticism, resilience, elastic power, speed, cognitive perceptual performance, and support. Let's get right into it!

1. Recovery

Recovery is one of the main tools in your performance arsenal. It is a natural process that can be very passive, but doesn't have to be. In order to allow for recovery, you must tap into a parasympathetic state of relaxation, the opposite of the fight or flight response. I've mentioned heart rate variability before — measuring it can help give you a lot of insight into your recovery. Additionally, don't forget to track the rate of perceived exertion and log it into your journal. This will also help you gauge your recovery. Beyond that, sleep, meditation, nutrition, and soft tissue work are all crucial elements of this tool. Members of your performance team can also give you specific advice for your situation. Be patient, recovery is an ongoing process! It's happening even when you're not thinking about it.

The following may seem like simple advice, but many people forget it: Do not underestimate the benefits of off-days. If you want to exponentially expedite your recovery, learn to know when to shut down for a day. Not everyone has this luxury, but if you are serious about recovery you need to plan vacation days in advance. In Major League Baseball, many teams have a predetermined amount of innings for a pitcher to throw before they automatically put them on some level of intermittent rest, regardless of how they feel. Taking time off will not only allow you to recharge your batteries, but will also allow you to pay attention to other areas of your life.

In general, when you are making decisions throughout your day, you should be viewing them through the lens of your recovery; is this alcoholic beverage or sweet snack going to hinder my recovery? Will staying up for a night on the town before a big workout the next day really allow me to get the most out of my session? Does a fight with my significant other allow myself to be in a relaxed state? The answer does not always need to lead to restricting yourself (we all need to let loose sometimes), just make sure to keep your recovery at the top of your mind so you do not get in the way of your own successful recovery process.

The Reset Breath is one form of a conscious breathing strategy to tap into a better physical and mental state by controlling your physiology which I covered in chapter 6. Here is another breathing method to serve your recovery. Diaphragmatic breathing is a conscious breathing technique which focuses on "belly breathing" rather than utilizing the accessory respiratory muscles throughout your upper body including your neck and chest. The diaphragm is a dome-shaped muscle which lies at the floor of your rib cage and flattens when it contracts. This muscle is one of the single most important muscles in terms of both respiration and spine health. A full diaphragmatic breath leads to an optimal amount of intra-abdominal pressure while also tapping into a more effective breath with less accessory muscle tension. In addition to your daily meditation practice where you might already be performing diaphragmatic breaths, there should be daily time devoted towards it. Think of this as centering your natural energy and activating your diaphragm, a most important core muscle which attaches to many different organs and muscles in and around your spine. More importantly, it puts you in a state of ultimate relaxation. No matter what injury you may have sustained, activating your diaphragm will have benefits. Having a stable base, by building an optimal amount of pressure in our abdominal cavity, will help the rest of our musculoskeletal system function properly.

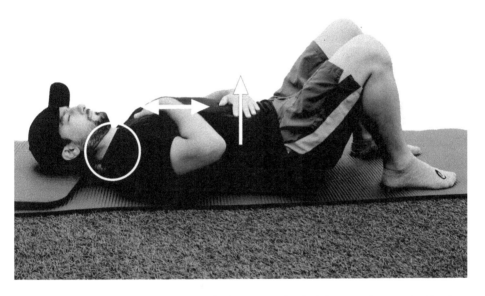

White circle emphasizes the need to keep a neutral neck while maintaining your shoulders in a relaxed position during the entire respiration cycle. Arrow along chest shows that you should aim to prevent your chest from significantly rising with the use of your top hand as feedback. Arrow at belly pointing up indicates where your belly should be rising during the respiration, using your hand as feedback.

Steps to Diaphragmatic Breathing

1. Laying on your back with your legs either bent, or resting on an elevated surface, place one hand on your chest and one hand on your stomach.
2. Begin by inhaling through your nose slowly counting *at least* five seconds without letting the hand on your chest rise, feeling the breath fill your abdomen in all directions. Avoid shrugging your shoulder or tightening your neck muscles.
3. Exhale through pursed lips (like blowing out a candle) slowly and completely until you empty your lungs. Towards the end of the breath you should feel your abdominals slightly contract. In some people the exhalation can take 2.5 times as long as the inhalation so don't be afraid to exaggerate the exhalation.
4. Perform at least five breaths in this manner at least once per day. This can also be performed in a seated position instead of on your back if that's more comfortable for you.

A subject related to recovery that you may be wondering about but that has not yet been discussed is soft tissue and manual work. This can include manual treatment, massage therapy, cupping, acupuncture, adjustments from a chiropractor, and self-treatment with a Theragun, foam roll, or other instrument-assisted soft tissue mobilization (IASTM) devices. Though, like much of the research in the field of performance, results on the use of manual soft tissue work have been highly inconclusive, ask any professional athlete (and many of my patients), and they will tell you about the time they got a magical massage or manual treatment which enhanced their recovery and/or performance.

Many of us clinicians become jaded by manual work because our clients and patients tend to become somewhat dependent on these treatments. And while providing them is good for the business end of a clinical practice, in the medical world our goal is to bill out and perform only necessary services. So when you are working in a professional team setting, or having a client ask for these extra services, it sometimes becomes a dilemma: Do we just give-in and do what the patient/client requests regardless of whether it's actually beneficial? In my practice, I have found that the best path is to educate athletes to where they feel like they can make an informed decision about their treatment options.

In a professional or collegiate sports athletic training room, it is not uncommon to hear this referred to as a "spa" day. In terms of recovery, these spa days do sometimes lead to the relaxation needed to get athletes over the hump of their recovery. But they can also be seen as similar to snacking when bored — an impulsive, rather than a rationally thought-out act. In your own recovery, consider: Do those muscles really need to be agitated at that moment? In that vein, the number one thing with any manual treatment, whether you are rolling on a foam roll or getting a massage, is to have a clear idea of the intended result, and how it addresses a finding within your musculoskeletal or neuromuscular assessment; if you are having a manual technique performed to your hip flexor then there should be a specific and objective measure that you're using to assess the pre- and post-work treatment. When you are working with a clinician, they should be experienced in the manual technique that they are using, and be able to clearly explain the process and result you should expect. All in all, my recommendation is that you use these services sparingly so that their effect will be greater when you really do need the work performed.

Proper measurement, days off, diaphragmatic breathing, and manual work are all helpful to recovery in their individual ways. Stay on track and build these techniques into habits during your Injured to Elite journey. They are all easy and potentially effective ways to streamline your recovery. Complicated doesn't mean better here, instead consistency is key.

2. Athleticism

Athleticism is a loaded term. While it can specifically refer to abilities related to sports, it doesn't at all have to. I have had clients whose explicit performance goals had nothing to do with athleticism in that way. Goals such as regaining the ability to engage in physical activities or demands such as hiking or sailing, or even being able to sit through a movie without pain put athleticism in a different context altogether. Let's face it, not everyone wants to become a professional athlete, which is just fine because my goal has always been to help high-performing athletes as well as individuals who have less conventional physical goals. As humans, we share the majority of DNA that makes up our physical body, and that idea is the basis for how we think of this tool; athleticism here, then, is not referring to the ability to run around defenders or perform a ladder drill better than someone else, but one's general level of physical preparedness as a human being.

We use general physical preparedness (GPP) as a fundamental training principle in the performance world referring to a baseline level of fitness and readiness that we all require before loading into more advanced levels of training. Deconditioning happens quickly after injury as I am sure you have felt already. Your level of general physical preparedness will almost certainly decline initially due to your limited activity status. That's why now is the time to quickly rebuild that general level of fitness considering the modifications based on your needs after injury. For instance, if you have an arm injury the focus will be on the legs, and the opposite for a leg injury. The goal is to get moving however you can as early as allowed. That said, you should work with your team to be deliberate about what you're doing. In the sports performance world, we say that loading bad movement patterns only enhances your weaknesses — a byproduct of working harder instead of smarter. There will always be a place for the grunt workout like when we need to mentally let off steam or increase our heart rate to wake our system up, but in the long haul we should strive for a relentless work ethic and be powered by an intelligent approach.

Allowing your injured area to naturally recover while reinforcing the rest of your system will put you in a better place than most right off the bat. For one thing, the rest of your body will give the injured area the opportunity to heal by being better able to pick up the slack. This fits in with some of the basic principles of athleticism and GPP, which encompass the ability to perform basic amounts of work that a human is expected to perform. For example, every athlete should be able to run a mile in a reasonable amount of time. It does not matter if you are an ultra-endurance athlete or a sprinter, the point is having a baseline level of cardiovascular fitness.

If you can run, shoot for an 8-minute mile. If you can't run yet, then use biking as a marker utilizing a 1:3 ratio of one mile running as roughly equivalent to three miles biking. If your lower half is under construction, then using a rowing machine or upper body ergometer to perform a few 500-meter sessions in less than three minutes with 30-60 second rest in-between can be a great alternative. All of these will demonstrate a good amount of baseline cardiovascular fitness. My point is for you to understand that no matter what your injury is, it is possible to regain and keep up a general level of fitness by creatively working around your injury. Note, this isn't about breaking personal records, but rather getting that baseline fitness you require to progress into more complex tasks.

Another area related to general physical preparedness is a baseline amount of range of motion and movement. Here, I recommend consulting with the appropriate performance team member in order to get some specific and objective range of motion findings. However, there are also some basic principles you can easily learn on your own starting with using your own eyes with a mirror or video to assess your movements.

Gray Cook is the founder of the Functional Movement System (FMS), which utilizes a movement screen that looks at seven different movement patterns. During my time with the Cardinals, I became certified in the FMS and SFMA (Selective Functional Movement Assessment). Think of when you go for your yearly physical and your physician asks you to perform physical tasks such as standing on one leg and touching your nose. Movement screens such as this allow performance professionals to look at the overall quality of movement to determine potential imbalances, weaknesses, and stability issues that might need further evaluation. This information can help modify training regimens to decrease risk of injury and to improve quality of movement that can help to optimize overall performance. A simple analogy is when the wheel alignment is off on a car, the tires wear out unevenly and sometimes more quickly. When a specific and basic movement is uneven, unsteady, or downright poor, this can cause parts of your body to experience higher levels of stress. It might not be an issue when you're just focusing on walking your dog down the block, just like you might not notice your wheel alignment is off when driving a short distance to grab some groceries, but take the car on the highway for 50 miles, or try running a few miles and boom! All of a sudden the deficit becomes magnified! That is why we try and work on evaluating the quality of your movement before pushing past your current limits.

The FMS is certainly not an end-all be-all screen, however it is one of the most widely-used and researched screens out there. Basically, the lower your score on it, the higher your risk of injury. I am not proposing that you become an expert in the FMS, rather that you learn some simple self-assessment concepts in order for you to be able to start evaluating how you are moving. Just a few of the FMS-based movement assessments like the overhead squat, push-up, in-line lunge, and active straight leg raise, can tell you a lot about your general movement quality.

Movement Self-Assessment Crash-Course

There are many ways for you to gain insight into your movement patterns, but perhaps the most effective way is to simply record your basic movements with a mobile device. Even just assessing your squat, leg raise, pushup, and overhead arm raise, can potentially tell you a tremendous amount about the quality of your overall movement. While I recommend discussing these movements with your team, I also encourage you to take some ownership here and learn some basics of assessment for yourself. When you know yourself, those helping you will be in an even better position to offer you empowering guidance!

Here is a list of things that we look for universally when assessing movement to get you started on your own self-assessment research:
- ◆ Control and steadiness of the movement
  - ○ Is the movement smooth or jerky?
- ◆ Alignment
  - ○ Are joints kept in neutral positions?
- ◆ Range of Motion
  - ○ Can the individual complete a full movement?

Now that you have an idea of a few qualitative elements that us professionals are looking at when we ask you to walk down the catwalk in the PT office and perform other repetitive movements, let's dive deeper into a few basic areas of movement.

I am going to break down each basic movement or physical ability and discuss ways for you to understand it. Remember, though this book is not written to work with your specific physical obstacle, these are all general principles that can apply to most individuals. This is a mostly agnostic approach to assessing and optimizing your own physical movement regardless of your background. If you do have the ability to work on this, then I recommend you do so, as long as it doesn't go against the recommendations of your own clinicians! In fact, feel free to share and discuss this with them, since there are often differences in how people interpret details, not to mention that they can advise you on any modifications needed based on your specific history. Remember, along with your own experience (and research), evidence-based medicine also relies on the experiences of us clinicians.

Postural Stability: First up is postural stability because without this, the rest of our movements would inevitably suffer. Postural stability is our ability to maintain optimal alignment throughout our body's joints during specific positions, especially when upright, although it applies to other bodily positions as well. The term "postural stability" relates to maintaining alignment during a movement and while at rest. The parts of our body that are central to this include our pelvis, neck, shoulders and feet. I suggest initially working on learning how to find the neutral positions for all of these in a way that is most appropriate for you. This can be standing, sitting, or lying down on your back (supine).

Neutral Pelvis: Start with your hands on your hips rocking back and forth going from a position where the curve in your lower back goes from fully rounded to fully arched, finding the midpoint of both extremes. We call this position neutral pelvis, and it is where you should ideally maintain at rest and when performing most movements.

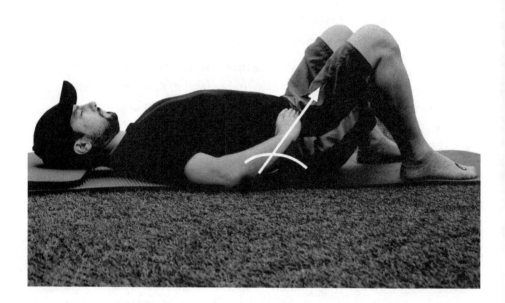

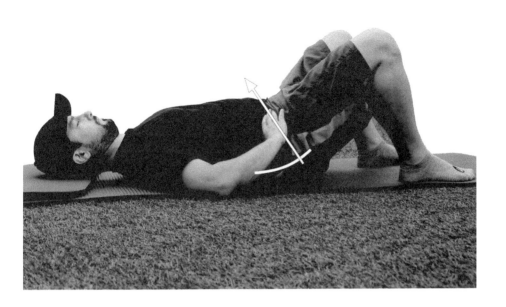

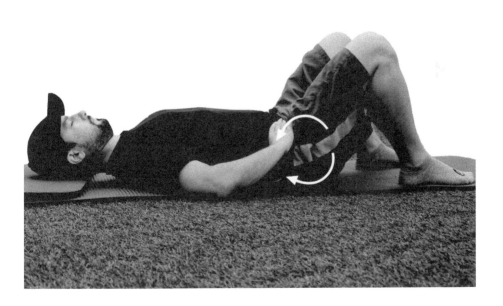

Neutral Neck: Your ear should be in-line with your shoulders, avoiding the undesirable forward head posture. This is specifically important when working on a computer, when using our mobile devices, and even driving. Simply find this by placing a finger on your chin and going back and forth into full protraction and retraction of the neck (cervical spine) simulating the clucking of a chicken. There should remain a slight curve or arch in the back of your neck. It may feel like you are in a neutral neck position when in fact you are really still quite out of alignment especially when just learning this, so I would suggest using a mirror.

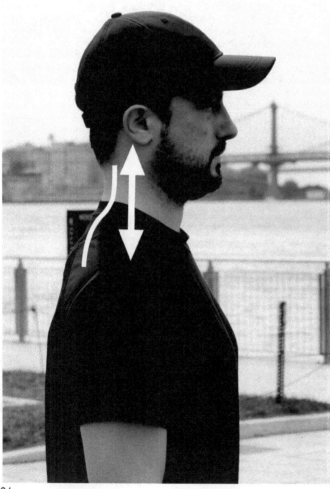

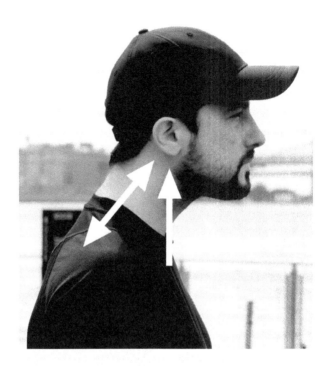

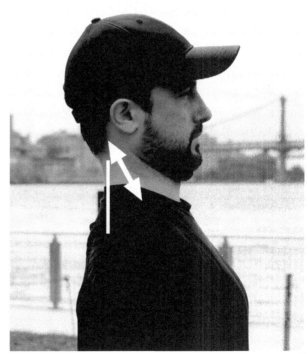

Neutral Foot: So most of us have considered whether we have a low or high arch. Not only is the whole shoe industry interested in foot posture but so are performance professionals who are looking to optimize movement. Foot anatomy is quite complex, as I learned during my doctoral training, especially during a clinical experience where my instructor had me walking around with a foot/ankle model for the first week. Regardless of the complexity, what I would like you to know here is that just as with the neck and pelvis, a more neutral arch is ideal. There are injuries associated with both a high arch (such as ankle sprains) and a low arch (such as different types of tendinitis). Vladimir Janda (1928-2002), a Czechoslovakian physician who was an expert in posture, came up with the Janda Short Foot Exercise, which has had tremendous influence in the world of physical rehabilitation. The exercise essentially activates the intrinsic foot muscles including the arches of the feet. While it is easy to mistake this for simply raising your arch, this movement is a bit more complex.

Start in a lesser weight bearing position such as sitting with your feet pointing straight ahead hip-width apart on the floor. Imagine that there is a string from the tip of your toes to your heel that you are attempting to shorten, hence the name of the exercise titled "short foot." Now go ahead and tighten the deep muscles of the foot slightly "shortening" the foot while activating the bottoms of your arch. It is a very subtle movement but the most important key is not to lift the base of your big toe off of the ground as this is the usual compensation we see with this exercise. This will benefit everything above your foot by allowing for a more stable connection to the ground, enhancing the rest of your movement and force through the ground. It can take stress off of other areas of your body that might be exerting effort to dissipate forces from the ground.

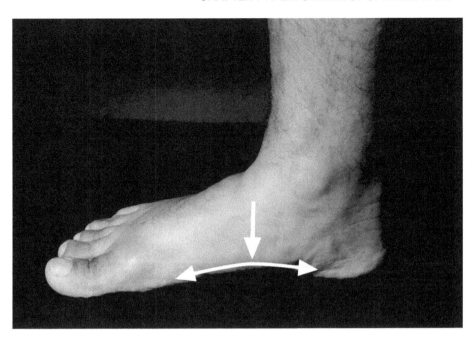

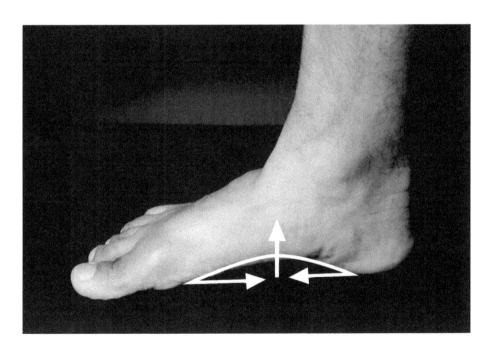

Neutral Shoulder: The baseball rehab guy always gets asked questions about the shoulder and elbow! Yup, that was me! The truth is we don't need to be pitchers or throwing athletes to think about our shoulder positioning. As a matter of fact, physical therapists see a good amount of shoulder injuries in non-athletic populations; it just so happens that, due to its anatomy, the ball and socket shoulder joint is rather unstable to start. This instability allows for more movement in all directions, but it comes at the cost of a higher injury risk. Even if you are not a baseball player, I bet at some point you've wondered why your shoulders were feeling so tight. It has even become the quintessential area we expect a massage when someone offers! There are a ton of big muscle attachments to the four joints that make up our shoulders, and they tend to do a lot of work to maintain the level of stability and movement we desire from our upper body. Go ahead and follow along with a few of these concepts on shoulder posture.

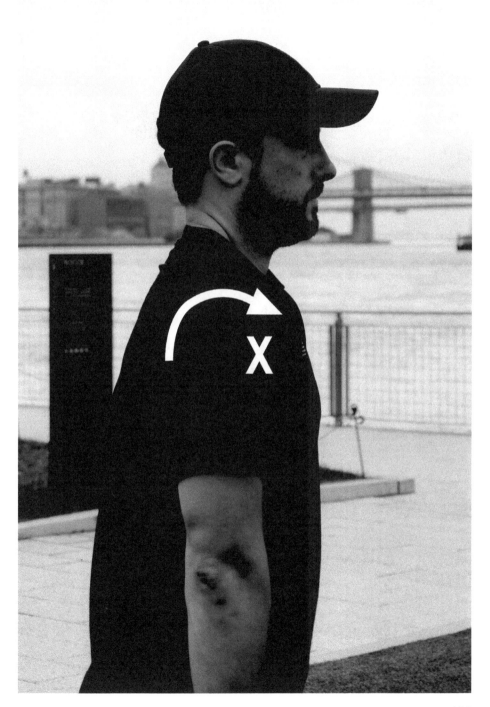

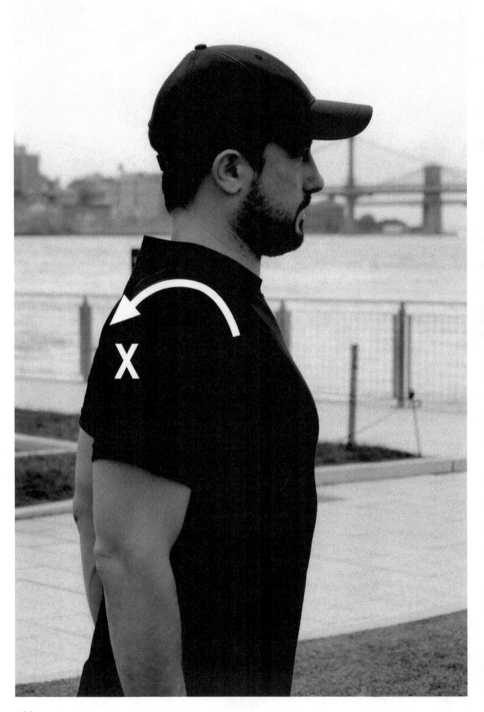

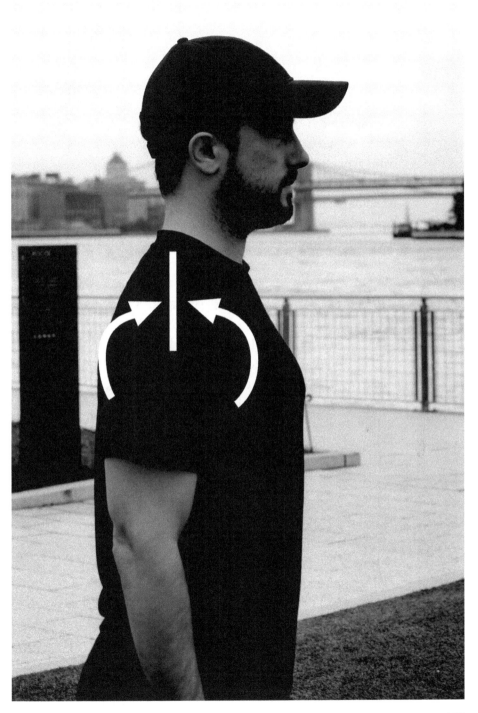

1. Shoulders should be even when looking in the mirror! If one is significantly higher than the other work on finding an even shoulder height (note, it can be like a chicken or the egg problem in determining which side is too high or too low, so just choose the one that feels right). Usually we hadn't even realized that one shoulder was significantly higher and all it took was the visual cue to correct the imbalance. When this doesn't seem to correct things, I recommend digging deeper with your clinician. Remember, this isn't just about your resting posture, so also pay attention to the location of your shoulder blades when you are performing other movements as well. Do you have a tendency to tighten up more on one side than the other and elevate your shoulder blade? If so, this can be a great thing to work on in order to optimize your shoulder postural stability.

2. The next thing to think about is keeping our shoulders in good overall alignment with the rest of our midsection. Many of us have been told not to round our shoulders, but have you ever been told to keep your shoulder blades back? Well, that can sometimes be poor guidance as over-"pinching" our shoulder blades can take our upper extremities out of ideal alignment as well. The reason being that our muscles operate on an ideal length/tension relationship, and holding our shoulder blades too far back can throw that out of whack. Here, we want to find neutral again by doing a shoulder roll all the way forward and then backward, eventually leaving them in the middle of those two extremes. If you see a pattern developing in these descriptions, it's clear that doing these simple exercises can become a nice reset for the body. Just as you learned the reset breath to regulate your breathing, emotions, and mindset, these are the ways to reset your body positioning. Remember we aren't talking about keeping these positions at all times but rather using them as tools to get to the ideal positions.

3. Ideal shoulder blade positioning in relationship to the rib

cage and spine is the last important element of finding your neutral shoulder position. This also happens to be the most difficult part of your body to adjust because the shoulder blades are difficult to visualize (since they're behind your body), as well as serving as free-floating bones. For this, you will likely have to use a more weight-bearing position for the upper extremity to train properly. The exercise requires you to get on all fours. While on your hands and knees, your hands should be shoulder-width apart and your knees hip-width apart. Keeping your elbows straight push the ground away with your hands raising your trunk towards the ceiling. Go back and forth (still keeping the rest of your spine in position) finding the position where your shoulder blades are fully flush with your rib cage and your trunk is maximally pushed towards the ceiling. Work on finding and holding this position starting with just 5-10 seconds for a few sets. Don't worry about finding this while standing or during other movements, but rather just use this exercise to work on your overall shoulder blade stability.

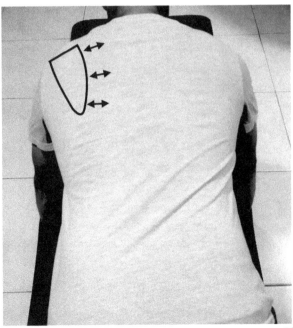

"Normal" Walking Gait and Other Forms of Locomotion: Our walking pattern and other forms of locomotion (wheelchair ambulation, crawling, etc.) can tell us a lot, including our overall level of recovery. Perhaps you are unable to walk at all due to a severe injury and were prescribed an assistive device or some other form of durable medical equipment such as a wheelchair or crutches to help you with your overall mobility. This also includes those who might have had a tough training session the day before and are now limping around, sometimes unknowingly. It also includes those that are showing a negative emotional state through body language! It is no coincidence why tons of class time for us physical therapists is spent learning about human gait patterns. Gait patterns are something very unique to the human experience, from the mind all of the way down to injury. Indeed, this overlooked area in the sports performance world can give us a lot of insight. For those that are reliant on forms of locomotion other than walking, there are amazing professionals out there who are adept at educating you on optimizing your movement. That said, many of the above principles should still hold true for you.

In episode 13 of *The Injured to Elite* podcast, celebrity DJ Mateo Difontaine shares his story of losing his leg to a flesh-eating bacterial infection known as necrotizing fasciitis. This condition left him having to learn how to walk in a new way with the use of a prosthetic lower extremity, though he oftentimes uses a wheelchair to get around due to the convenience it can offer. We are talking about a man who still surfs with some famous big wave surfers using his artifical leg (*cough* *cough* John *cough* Denney *cough* *cough*). But in the episode, Mateo explained to me how on certain days he just doesn't want to get into the wheelchair and how this gives him a sense of dread. Our ability to be independent and mobile, whether we are walking with our own two legs or using an assistive device, is an experience that is deeply felt by us on an emotional level as human beings. After all, why go from injured to elite if for no other reason than to be mobile in our world? Neglect looking at your way of getting around, or gait pattern, and risk not going to that elite level I know you desire.

If you find that you are unable to walk utilizing a normal gait pattern and require modifications, don't let that discourage you from your journey. Successful athletes go through journeys that involve wheels, crutches, artificial limbs, or canes, and come out on the other end with a healthy mind and body (even if it continues to involve these assistive devices). Whatever it takes, I recommend you spend time with someone who can really help you get the most out of whatever you are using to help yourself get around. Oftentimes, it is best to find a specialist, but don't be afraid to mastermind the process with a more generalized clinician. Physical therapists, for example, can be very creative in coming up with strategies to help anyone and everyone. For those fortunate enough to use your own two legs, below are some important points to think about in terms of a normal gait pattern.

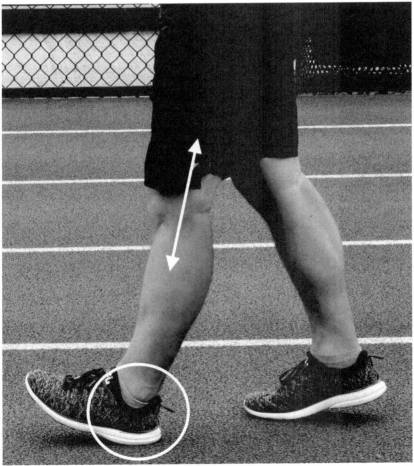

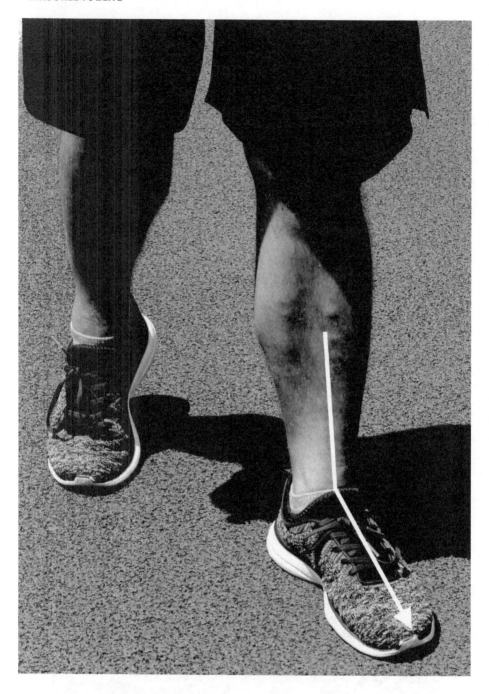

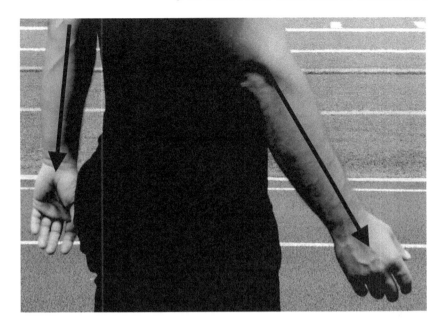

1. There is no "perfect" walk: As a matter of fact, a former PT colleague of mine pointed out that I tend to hyper-extend my knees when I walk! I don't mind and neither does my body.

2. There is a difference between relearning your normal walking pattern (gait) after injury or surgery, versus just going on long walks as a form of exercise. A lot of times I am asked by a patient after an injury if they should start walking more. I always tell them that before worrying about how much to walk, they should focus on relearning a healthy walking pattern. Then sure, walk your heart out! Indeed, walking is actually a great way to holistically work on your performance. It can be an effective low-impact exercise for the body since we are designed to walk, a great way to calm and renew the mind, and an ideal time to ponder our visions and dreams (more on this in part three). We can't always hit every one of those points during an intense training session, but when we walk there is plenty of time to do it all.

3. Here are a few very basic biomechanical considerations to think about especially when relearning how to walk after an

injury:

a. Generally, we should have a nice heel-toe gait pattern where our heel hits the ground first when taking a step forward.

b. When our heel hits the ground, our knee should be in a relatively straight position.

c. Maintain a modest stride length and be cautious not to overstride. When our foot is too far in front of our body for our base of support, our lower extremity muscles have less ability to absorb force.

d. When you push off your back foot it should be relatively straight in order to evenly distribute weight through the foot and lower extremity. If you find yourself turning your toes far inward or outward, work on improving your overall foot alignment during your gait.

e. Lastly, to wrap up the gait section, remember it is very important to think about the other joints of the body. When we walk our arms should swing in the opposite directions of our legs. We call this "reciprocal arm swing," and it helps us walk efficiently. Another part of the body to remember outside of just the lower extremities is the pelvic section. If you tend to oversway your hips while walking, that can lead to more shearing forces at your lower back and other areas. If that's the case, you should work on maintaining activation of your midsection and core even when walking. Careful not to overtighten, and just work on gently bracing outward with your stomach.

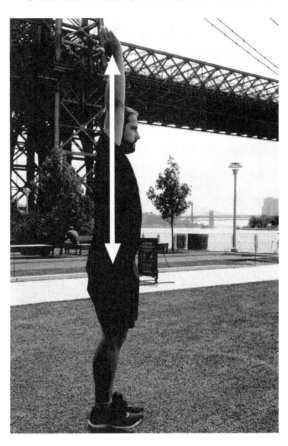

Overhead Movement: As I mentioned previously it's important for the shoulder joint to be flexible, yet still stay stable. Since we already covered the stability part let's move on to the easier part: Seeing if it is moving enough. Recording with your mobile device from a side angle, establish a standing position with your hands at your side, elbows straight, and thumbs out in front of you. While keeping your arm straight, elevate your arms fully overhead as high as you can go. Ideally, you are able to elevate your arm fully overhead so that your upper arm and bicep area is parallel to your ear. If you are a bit lower than this, that is not necessarily a problem, but it can be an area for you to address with shoulder mobility exercises such as performing some soft-tissue work with a small ball.

Below are a few common compensatory movements that we find in people that struggle to demonstrate a full range of motion with their shoulders:

◆ Over-arching of the mid-back and spine to help elevate the arms

◆ Forward head posture to cheat the way into the overhead movement

◆ Arms shift slightly to the side (more like a V or Y) rather than straight overhead

◆ Overall, we look to see that there is not excessive movement in the upper trapezius muscle (upper shoulder) that looks like a shrug. This is a very common compensation for those who have undergone shoulder surgery for their rotator cuff.

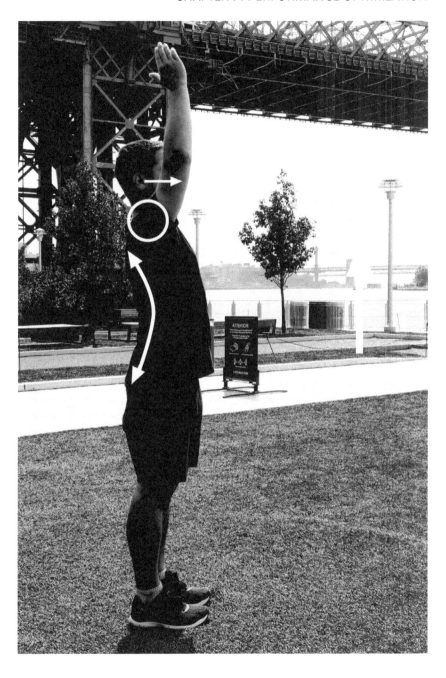

Corrective Movement for Lack of Overhead Flexion: If you find yourself lacking good overhead shoulder movement, my go-to "corrective exercise" when you're by yourself is using a ball to perform some tissue mobilization while going through an overhead movement. The ball works to "pin down" and stretch the tissue surrounding the back of the shoulder while the arm goes into an overhead movement. This can help to alleviate restrictions in movement by providing somewhat nociceptive (painful) acupressure to an area where the muscle is more tense, decreasing tone in the area and allowing for a greater range of motion. This combines principles of soft tissue work and motor control (it affects the nervous system rather than just stretching muscles).

Why is this exercise my most universally helpful corrective movement for overhead shoulder restriction? Because, as I mentioned before, it provides soft tissue mobilization while simultaneously going through a good quality movement pattern that is training the brain to go through a full arc of motion with little compensatory patterns. Sure, I have other, fancier methods to achieve these things but a major principle in this book is to teach and empower you to be able to do what you can on your own. That said, as a responsible medical professional, I will once again remind you that if you do have a shoulder restriction for whatever reason, please consult with a trusted member of your team before attempting this exercise.

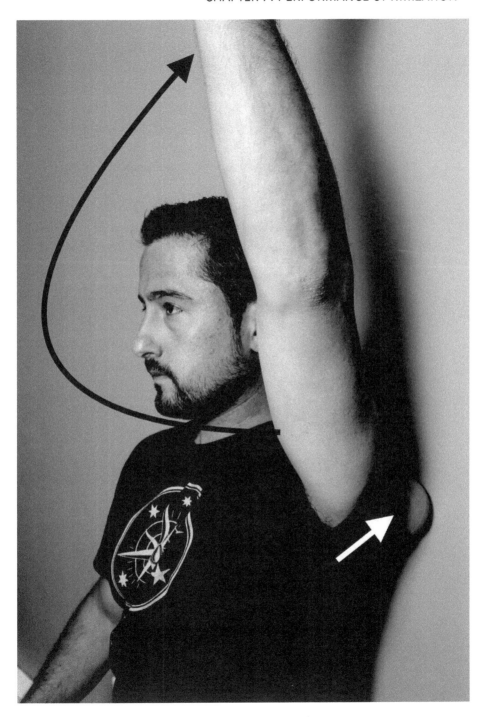

- ◆ Begin by spending 30-90 seconds (as time permits) applying moderate pressure with a small ball (think lacrosse or tennis ball) into the back of the shoulder where the muscular part behind the ball-and-socket joint meet the "lat" muscle as seen in the picture on the previous page. Pressure should be somewhat uncomfortable but still tolerable. Scan the area around the back of the shoulder as you roll the ball to find the tender spots and spend the 30-90 seconds holding pressure in those areas.

- ◆ Lift your arm in front of your body with thumbs pointing in front of you. If you were to perform this movement fully your upper arm should end several inches from the side of your ear.

- ◆ While performing a few repetitions of this movement (5-10) make sure to keep your upper trapezius (top of the shoulder muscle) nice and relaxed throughout the range of motion.

- ◆ Recheck your shoulder range of motion following this session just as initially performed. Sometimes there is a notable increase after doing it only once, while at other times you might not see a big difference right away. In those situations, it requires a few sessions.

Squat: Kind of like elite, squat is a charged word! People can misinterpret elite to mean something arrogant rather than high-performing, just like people can interpret a squat as a dangerous exercise that will almost certainly lead to a back injury. In reality, a squat is a basic movement pattern that we do on a daily basis such as when we go from a standing to seated position. Many times, an inability to demonstrate a quality squat pattern is related to control rather than weakness or flexibility, so often it just requires some special attention and practice rather than specific exercises. Depending on your individual situation, you might require a more intensive assessment and more specific programming, but the following instructions should still serve as a guide for you to drive your own movement improvements forward. Here is what you should know about assessing your ability to perform a squat:

1. This is a more knee-dominant versus hip-dominant movement, meaning that more load and motion occur at the knee joint rather than the hip joint. The more forward one's center of mass shifts the more knee-dominant the movement becomes. If the knees were to be past the toes, that would be too knee-dominant a movement, which we tend to suggest avoiding.

2. It is best to get a good sense of this movement from all angles; front, back, and each side. Here is what you are looking for in each view.
   a. Frontal view (anterior):
      i. An even weight distribution on both lower extremities without any significant weight shift onto one side, keeping even on both hips.
      ii. The ability to keep your knees in good alignment without them caving in or pushing outwards.
   b. Back view (posterior):
      i. Once again assess that your hips are even without a significant weight shift to either side. It can be particularly helpful assessing this from the back as you can get a better view of the spine and back of the pelvis.

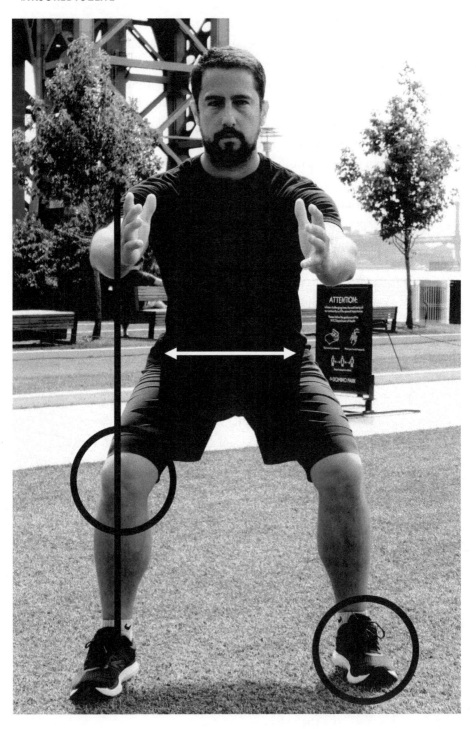

c. Side view (from both left and right):

   i. Your knees should ideally travel no further than the tip of your toes in order to avoid an overly knee-dominant movement with too high a stress applied to the front of the knee, although some research shows that this is, in fact, okay. A good way to ensure a balanced approach is by standing with your feet against a tall box, chair, or wall.

   ii. Look for a depth of movement where the thighs are able to move parallel to the floor.

Note: The squat will also be included in the following section with an emphasis on training and loading the pattern rather than assessing the movement.

Corrective Exercises, Mobility, Stability, and Motor Control

Part of your overall level of athleticism will be influenced by your movement patterns. If you or your team find impaired movements, you can implement specific corrective exercises, and modifications to the basic movements in your training program, to improve your baseline performance. There is a very fine line between a corrective exercise and a rehabilitation exercise — or as us physical therapists call it in our documentation, "therapeutic exercises." A corrective exercise is a specific exercise designed to improve an overall movement pattern or posture. This can be a stretch, movement, strengthening exercise, or a modification of another more conventional exercise. For example, if you have a limited amount of mobility in your ankle, this can affect your ability to perform a deep squat, and can also impact your sprinting technique. Performing an exercise to "correct" the ankle mobility and overall movement, such as kneeling on one knee and driving the opposite knee (of the restricted ankle) forward past your toes while holding onto a stick, focuses specifically on the issue in question.

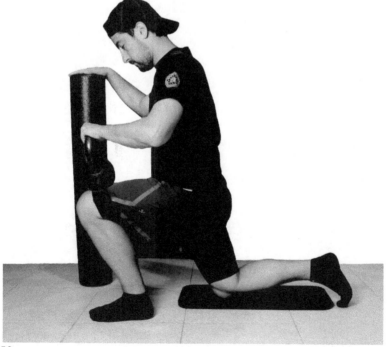

Every program should have at least a few corrective exercises based on your assessment findings. I recommend logging these findings into your own performance journal, and putting the exercises into your daily routine. Corrective exercises should be included in your general warm-up prior to both workouts and actual activities. These movements are not intended to fatigue your system but rather to prepare areas of the body for more intense and loaded movement. If you recall the activities scale that I suggested in the load management section, a corrective or rehab exercise should be a 3 out of 5 in terms of overall effort.

In working with a clinician and your own self-monitoring, the two of you should identify specific priority areas based on the assessment findings. There are three main types of priority areas for all parts of the body, they are mobility, stability, and motor control. Mobility and stability priorities are often confused with one another. Mobility is a general term for movement through a range of motion, whereas stability refers to the ability to maintain alignment either at rest or during a movement; in the latter, if something is off, you'll have difficulty keeping indirectly connected joints in your body steady. Commonly, my patients and athletes will report tightness and restriction in parts of their body that lack good stabilization. An example where mobility and stability are at odds is in a person who exhibits a ton of shoulder flexibility by being able to bring their arm into all positions (something we call joint laxity or hypermobility), yet lacks stability throughout the movements. This lack of stability might not be detected by the naked eye or even felt, however if one were to see what was going inside the joint, there could be "micro-instability" or poor centering of the bones within the joint throughout the range of motion.

The easiest way to think of the importance of stability is imagining a cannonball being shot out of a canoe. The boat would be very unstable leading to the cannonball taking a very short flight. The issue here is not power of the cannon or the balls ability to move through the air, but underlying stability of the whole setup. If the boat were to stay in a fixed and stable position such as off of a bigger boat anchored in the water, the ball would travel much further. It is important to understand that although you might feel that you are tight, weak, or moving poorly, the problem might be an underlying lack of stability around another part of the body. Our spine along with our ball-and-socket joints such as our hips and shoulders are the main areas where stability is needed for our extremities to move about freely; though you may feel tight in your hips or shoulders when attempting a movement, if the issue is stability rather than mobility, you are not correctly addressing the problem. In that case, I urge you to do more self-evaluation as well as working closely with your performance team to isolate the issues.

Motor control is a newer frontier in sports performance and refers to the ability of our entire nervous system to complete a desired physical movement or task. In certain situations while we may have good stability and mobility of a joint, we may still lack effective muscular firing patterns. Conveniently, this can be due to many factors that are already covered in this very book. For instance, pain and swelling can have a major impact on your ability to execute certain movements by limiting the nerve impulses in those areas. However, our nerves can be trained just like our muscles! As a matter of fact, most of the strength increases early on in a workout program are due to neuromuscular activation improvements. By waking up and better recruiting the nerves that serve our muscles, we're able to feel more competent in a movement.

If your performance team members have been keeping up with developments in sports performance then they will likely be very familiar with the importance of motor control. Motor control and stability have a lot of crossover but the main difference is that motor control looks at the movement as a whole, while stability is usually assessed joint by joint. If an athlete demonstrates a poor technique when squatting, their poor motor control may be a result of contributing stability and mobility issues. It's best not to guess, however — figuring out the root cause of the poor technique requires a thorough assessment by a knowledgeable professional. In writing that, I realize that I am not giving this topic nearly enough detail to make you an expert. My purpose, instead, is to make you aware of it so you can better discuss it with your team. Hopefully, they're familiar with it, though I am always surprised at the amount of professionals that do not understand this important concept.

Understanding this terminology puts you way ahead of the game, empowering you to understand how to better optimize your performance now and throughout your life. When troubleshooting an issue, you might ask yourself: Am I having mobility, stability, or perhaps a motor control issue? Then, you can ask this to your team members and be sure that the information you receive will be much more meaningful. It is after an injury, when you are increasing your overall athleticism and general physical preparedness and when you must modify more of your routine, that is the right time to build the proper foundation when it comes to developing proper movement patterns.

Workload Capacity and Change of Direction

Overall athleticism will depend on your workload capacity, and ability to quickly change directions. A great training and assessment tool for conditioning both your ability to increase your workload capacity, and change of direction is the 300 yard shuttle and the 5-10-5 Pro Agility Drill. Workload capacity and ability to quickly change directions put an athlete in an optimal position to demonstrate their skills. Even a non-traditional athlete can benefit from this; for example, they will be able to hike a long distance without experiencing significant fatigue, and/or be able to avoid obstacles during the hike. Pending that you are cleared by your medical professional and performance team members to begin this activity, here are the two drills, described briefly:

1. **300-Yard Shuttle:**
   One of the most widely used tests in collegiate and professional sports is the 300-yard shuttle run, or better known as 300s. This is a common training session in football, using the width of a football field (around 50 meters). Regardless of whether you have a football field available, you can place cones or place marks around 50

153

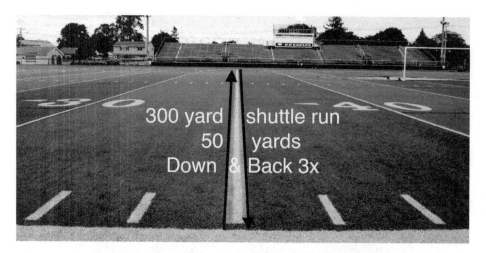

yards apart. Starting at one side you will run 50 yards straight across to the other cone and back on the same line, three times back-and-forth (no rest between laps), which will be a total of 300 yards. The goal is to complete this in less than one minute (as close as possible to 50 seconds). Once you become proficient in this, attempt to complete multiple 300-yard shuttles with two-minute rest intervals, while still aiming for a time of less than one minute per 300-yard set.

2. 5-10-5 Pro Agility:

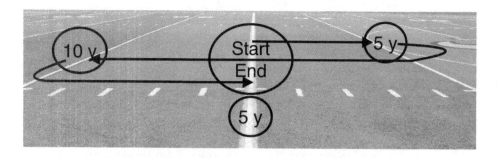

This drill is actually part of the National Football League's Annual Combine where incoming collegiate players that will potentially be drafted are tested. The athlete begins in the center of three cones or lines which are each five yards apart, hence the numbers 5-10-5. First the athlete runs five yards to the right, then quickly changes directions back to the left, running a full ten yards to the cone or line on the opposite side before finally returning the five yards to the right and through the starting point. A score of five seconds or below demonstrates a high-level division one collegiate athlete. You can perform several repetitions of this exercise with a rest:work ratio of about 4:1 — meaning if you are that collegiate athlete running it in five seconds, you would be resting at a minimum of 20 seconds between repetitions. The drill should be performed in both directions as an exercise allowing for balance and symmetry.

Note that although the lines in the photo are one above the other, the drill should be performed on the same path in all directions — a "straight shot" back and forth. As a caution, please be careful not to slam on the brakes when finishing this drill as this can lead to lower extremity injury, especially to the hamstrings.

3. Resilience

Resilience refers to our body's ability to withstand and recover quickly from both internal and external stresses. In order to build resilience past our baseline, we need to load specific fundamental movement patterns. The fundamental elements of any training program, regardless of the sport or activity or goal, should include a hinge, squat, and a bilateral push and pull, unilateral push and pull-based movement for both the upper and lower body. I have heard of just about every workout split you can imagine and have tried many of them myself. When I was 16 years-old and just beginning to work out with weights, I had my own performance journal and followed a bodybuilding-style routine, saving a specific day for biceps, etc. To put it lightly, my workout splits have evolved drastically over the years after immersing myself in dozens of different types of workout routines. My focus has become functionality over aesthetics, and I challenge those that want to perform at elite levels (not just look "elite") to go down this same path.

For those of you excited to get bigger, faster, and stronger, don't jump the gun yet thinking about Olympic-style lifting routines that include clean and jerks, or the newest CrossFit program. I have nothing against either of these practices as long as you have worked diligently at developing overall resilience, building a solid foundation by loading basic movement patterns. Since this book is a guide, not a specific workout recipe, I am not looking to share every exercise possible, but rather inspire you to creatively come up with a program that will be effective for you under the guidance of your team members. You can do it; though my colleagues and I do occasionally get so deep into our craft that we like to think it is— this isn't rocket science.

Training Fundamental Movements

Moving on, the key to building up tissue tolerance and overall resilience is to progressively load nine fundamental movements over time. During this process, there comes a moment when rehabilitation becomes training. More specifically, when your routine starts to look like the movements later in this chapter, you're getting close to the threshold. In this section, I will show you the return-to-activity process through fundamental movements that should comprise part of your strength-training regimen prior to making your full return.

First, there are a few terms that you should familiarize yourself with, so the descriptions of movement patterns make more sense. We refer to utilizing both left and right sides of the body as a *bilateral movement*, and utilizing one side of the body as a *unilateral-based movement*. Later, you will see examples of both bilateral and unilateral movement patterns for the upper and lower body. This will serve as the framework of your training.

Before going further, a few points about the movements in this section. First off, each of these movement patterns serve as a framework for many potential variations within that pattern. For example, a pushup is an example of a bilateral-based upper body pushing movement pattern. This does not, however, mean that you must specifically perform pushups as part of your program; if you were to decide against incorporating a normal pushup into your routine, there are plenty of other bilateral upper body push alternatives such as a wall pushup or a barbell bench press. If you get lost in trying to manage the gaps in your program, it is a good idea to consult with your team members since they should have expertise in the topic. Still, even if you do that, don't feel like you can't own the process yourself. To start, ask yourself: Which potential loaded exercises that fall within this overall movement pattern would be best for my current needs? Whether you choose one or more exercises is up to you — you can certainly program in days that include different variations, or have a goal to progress into those movements at a later time.

Next, I would like to share with you how many of us performance professionals insert core activation and training within a workout that may not include conventional crunches or planks. You learned earlier how a simple diaphragmatic breathing exercise can train your core, and the following is going to further increase your ability to more optimally train your overall stability. Unilateral exercises are just as important when it comes to training individual areas of the body as they are to the core. Whenever we are performing a pushing or pulling-based movement with only one side of our body in an unsupported fashion, our trunk stabilizers must activate in order to prevent the body from collapsing or rotating. In the sports performance world, we call this an anti-rotation based movement, hence where the core comes in. A commonly performed anti-rotation movement is the Palloff press, which is illustrated on the next page.

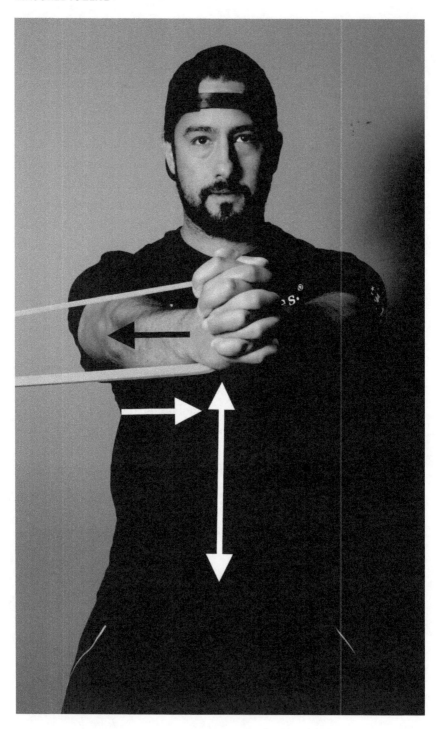

As the tension of the band is pulling my trunk and arms, I must activate my core stabilizers to prevent any rotation from occurring.

The other reason why unilateral work is beneficial can be understood with the following example: Let's say your right arm is weaker than your left due to an injury. If you were to perform a bilateral-based pushing movement such as a pushup, the overall movement pattern will be limited by the weaker side (in layman's terms, you'd be compensating and doing lopsided pushups). Therefore, unilateral work would allow you to appropriately adjust the workload ratio to properly benefit each side of the body.

Workload ratios can get quite complex, so my advice aims to simplify this process. Generally, I utilize unilateral-based exercises at a ratio of 1.5x more on the weaker side to help improve the balance. It makes sense then that, although you are improving the overall balance, you should expect that your body might react with more-than-usual soreness on that side. The variety of thinking behind unilateral workload ratios can probably become a book in themselves, but I'll summarize here with a few key take-home points:

♦ In addition to building resilience, you can also utilize unilateral training in order to better assess your strengths, weaknesses, and overall balance side-to-side.

♦ Remember that our side dominance or "laterality" is oftentimes a function of habit and daily life demands, so it is important to know why there is an imbalance first and foremost, since an imbalance is not always a bad thing. For that reason, before going forward with addressing the imbalance, get an idea of why it exists and if it is actually necessary to change.

♦ Determine how much to train the stronger side after first finding the appropriate amount of load (resistance/weight) and volume (sets, repetitions, rest intervals) by using the aforementioned 5-point graded activity scale (a corrective movement or rehab exercise is a 3/5, or moderate effort, whereas training or loading a body part in your regular workout is a 4/5, and performance enhancement, such as increasing power, is a 5/5)

◆ To reiterate, once the above step is completed a good rule of thumb to maintain balance in the body is to train the weaker side 1.5x the stronger side, or simply training the stronger side around 70% the amount of the weaker side. It might sound confusing, but the basic recommendation is to train the stronger side less. Again, this is for principles of balance, not necessarily for overall performance.

Earlier in this chapter you were taught how to assess and improve some of your postural positions, and important movements (the squat and overhead elevation of your upper extremities). Now you are going to learn the specific patterns of movement that you should be utilizing progressive resistance exercise with, in order to build up overall physical resilience. What you have learned thus far will carry over and even overlap into the section following that outlines the basic elements of any training program with strength in mind.

Before finally getting into the movement patterns to include in your workouts, I want to note the format it will be in. I will break down movements for the upper and lower body including bilateral and unilateral pushing and pulling movements. The reason why I will not be isolating particular muscles is that fundamental movement patterns include movement at multiple joints simultaneously, requiring the recruitment of many muscles, rather than just in isolation. We refer to this as a compound movement. For each movement pattern, proper alignment will be illustrated along with the commonly performed mistakes. I will also include a few regressions or progressions (lesser or increased load) for each of these movements to be seen instead based on your needs. Please also note that there is debate about some of the regressions/progressions, but this is to serve as a very general framework to give yourself guidance. Many of these movements can also include a vertical or horizontal line of pull variation, in terms of resistance.

Here are the nine fundamental patterns of movement along with specific suggested exercises that should be incorporated into your strength-training regimen to improve your tissue resilience:

1. Hinge
2. Squat
3. Lunge
4. Unilateral Hip Dominant Movement: Single-Leg Romanian Deadlift (RDL)
5. Bilateral Upper Body Pull: Reverse Pull-Up (with straight bar)
6. Bilateral Upper Body Push: Pushup (normal, ground-based)
7. Unilateral Upper Body Pull: Staggered Stance, Bent-over, Unilateral Row
8. Unilateral Upper Body Push: Staggered Stance Unilateral Push (Landmine Press)
9. Carry: Unilateral Farmer's Carry

You can use the following objects (or implements) for load:
◆ Household objects like textbooks or book bag
◆ Ankle/wrist weight
◆ Resistance band
◆ Weighted vest
◆ Weighted ball
◆ Dumbbell
◆ Kettlebell
◆ Barbell

Hinge

Lower Body: Bilateral Movement Patterns

Hip-Dominant

Illustration shows the middle portion of the movement starting fully upright.

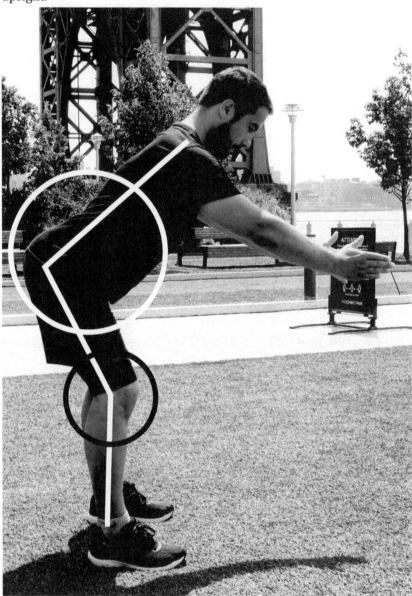

Proper Technique: The white line shows good alignment in the spine with a slight arch in the lower back (which is normal) and very slight rounding of the upper back. The larger circle shows that the hinge position is a hip-dominant movement. The lower circle shows that the knee is kept relatively straight during the movement.

Variations of this movement (from easier to challenging): Hinge with stick along spine, Standing Bilateral Anterior Reach with Hinge (as seen), Standing Banded Pull-Throughs, Standing RDL with weight off elevated surface, Suitcase RDL, Straight Bar RDL.

Poor Technique:

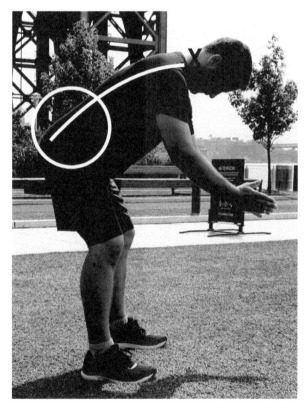

The X marks the common mistake of not maintaining a neutral neck position looking further downwards. The curved white line shows the lack of a neutral spine and the circle specifically highlights the rounding of the lower back. Aim to maintain a slight curve (arch) in the lower back.

Squat

Lower Body: Bilateral Movement Patterns

Knee-Dominant

The squat is a knee-dominant movement since the movement occurs with more motion and load at the knee joint rather than the hip as in hip-dominant movements. The vertical black line shows the legs slightly wider than shoulder width. The white arrow shows level hips, and the larger black circle on the right knee shows a neutral knee position. The smaller black circle on the left foot and ankle shows a relatively neutral position of the toes, although they can slightly point outwards.

Variations of this movement (from easier to challenging): Rocking Back and Forth on All 4's, Leg Press, Mini Squat with Hand Held Support on Surface of Object in front such as a chair, Sit to Stand off Chair, Free Body Weight Squat as seen, Front Loaded Squat, Back Loaded Squat, Overhead Squat.

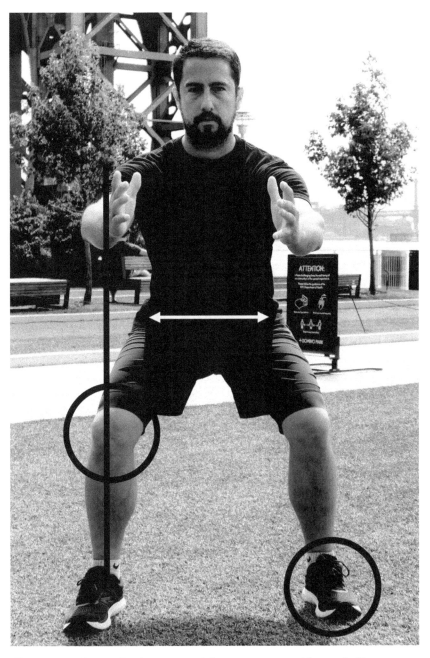

Illustration shows the first 30% of the movement with good alignment.

Poor Technique:

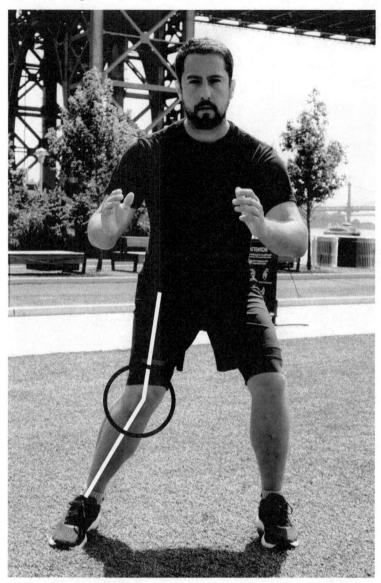

The circle on the right knee shows it collapsing into "dynamic valgus" (caving inward). This puts the lower extremity in overall poor alignment which can increase the stress on certain ligaments and parts of the foot, ankle, knee, hip, and spine. The feared ACL injury actually commonly occurs in an exaggerated, yet similar, position as seen above.

Lunge

Lower Body: Unilateral Movement Patterns

Knee-Dominant

Illustration shows the descent into a lunge with good alignment.

The circle in the middle of the image along with the arrow pointing downward shows good positioning of the hips within the middle of the base of support between my front and back foot. The white line along my shin indicates a relatively vertical shin angle, and lastly, the arrow in front of my right lower leg shows how my knee is staying behind the front of my toes allowing for decreased stress at the right knee cap "patella."

Variations of this movement (from easier to challenging): In-line Lunge with Hand Held Support on Foam Roll, Reverse Lunge with Band Assistance, In-line Lunge (as seen), Reverse Lunge, Step Up, Front Lunge, Split squat, Side Lunge

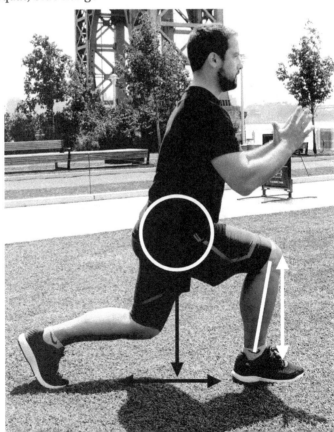

Poor Technique:

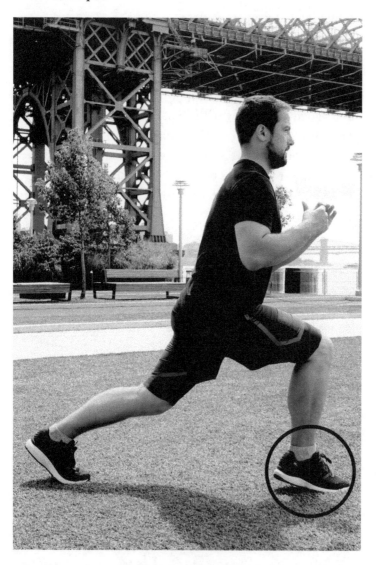

The circle around the right foot and ankle shows the common mistake made during lunge variations when failing to get the heel fully flat to the ground.

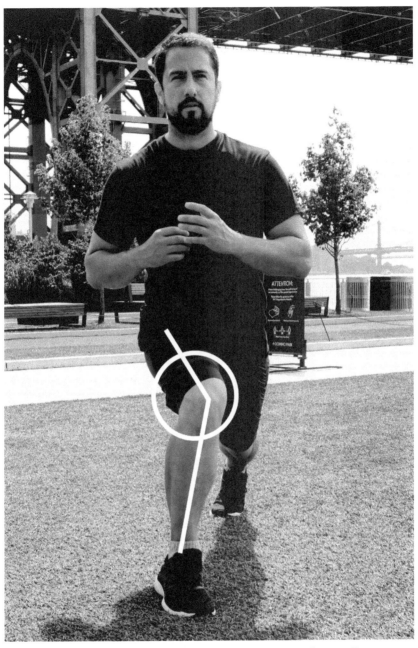

The lines and circle show the right knee falling into valgus collapse similar to the aforementioned Squat error.

Single-Leg RDL

Lower Body: Unilateral Movement Patterns

Hip-Dominant

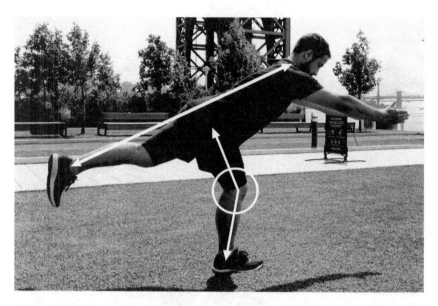

Illustration shows the descent down into a Single-Leg RDL with good alignment.

A Single-Leg RDL can be thought of as a single-leg hinge pattern movement. This is a more advanced movement since it requires a high degree of hip and trunk stability. Notice how the long straight arrow along the back of the body shows a relatively neutral spine and back leg. The arrows and circle along the right leg indicate a relatively straight right knee, however a slight bend in the knee is fine.

Variations of this movement (from easier to challenging): Holding onto wall with opposite side of leg and performing Bodyweight Single Leg Anterior Reach, holding onto wall with the same side of leg and performing Bodyweight Single Leg Anterior Reach, Single Leg Anterior Reach (as seen), Single Leg Anterior Reach with Band Resistance on

Opposite Side of Leg, Single Leg Anterior Reach with Band Resistance on Same Side of Leg, Single-Leg RDL with weight in both hands, Single-Leg RDL with weight in opposite hand, Single-Leg RDL with weight in same hand.

Poor Technique:

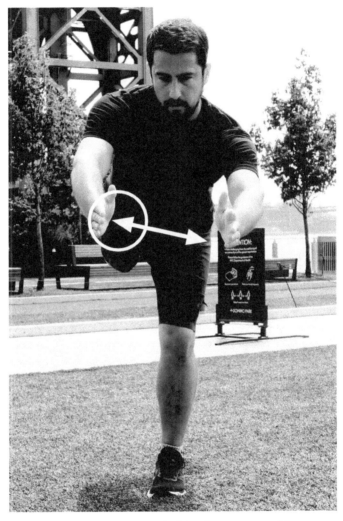

The white arrow and circle around my right hip show uneven hips elevated on the right. It is important to maintain even hip height throughout the movement, imagining that you are keeping the "headlamps" of your hips straight ahead.

Reverse Pullup with Straight Bar

Upper Body: Bilateral Movement Patterns

Pull

Illustration shows proper pull through around ½ the full range of motion with good alignment, starting fully upright.

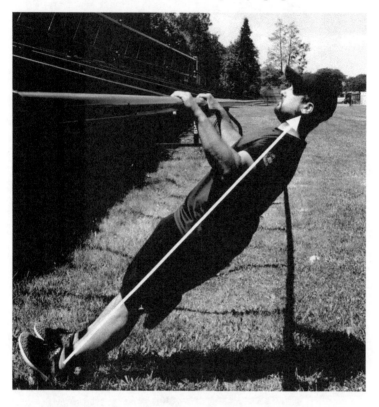

I find that this exercise is a nice antagonist movement to the classical bilateral-based pushing movement soon to follow, the pushup. This is a great way to promote symmetry especially when programming your exercises from a pushing and pulling standpoint. The white line above indicates great alignment from the ankles all the way up through the ear. Notice that the upper trapezius muscle (top of shoulders) appears relaxed along with a neutral position of the neck. The elbows are tracking out at a 45-degree angle with a relatively neutral wrist positioning.

Variations of this movement (from easier to challenging): Seated Mid Row with band or bar, TRX Row, Reverse Pull Up (as seen), Bent Over Barbell Row, Band Assisted Pull Up, Normal Pull Up.

Poor Technique:

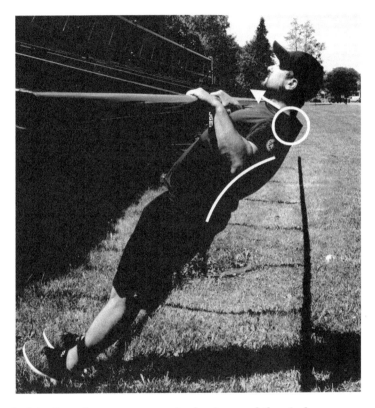

The curved white line shows an overarched spine, and the circle indicates over-activated upper shoulder (upper trapezius) muscles.

Normal Ground-Based Pushup

Upper Body: Bilateral Movement Patterns

Push

Illustration shows proper push through around ½ the full range of motion with good alignment.

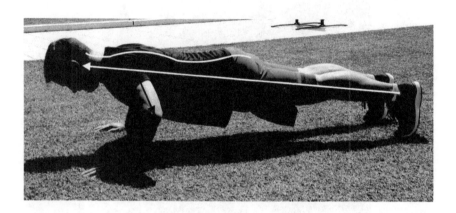

Who doesn't love a good pushup!? Okay, maybe plenty of you out there but we all remember being commanded or at least asked to do a pushup once in our life, right? How many times were you closely taught how to perform a good pushup? I bet many of you will answer none... For this reason, please note above some key points to performing a solid pushup. The white arrow demonstrates good trunk stability without any "lag" in the spine during the movement. The spine should have its normal curve as it depicted with the curved white arrow, a slight arch in the lower back and a slight rounding in the upper/mid back, with another slight arch in the neck. The black arrow shows the plane of movement for the elbow to track at around a 45-degree angle.

Variations of this movement (from easier to challenging): Wall Pushup, Incline Surface Pushup (on a table or bed), Modified Kneeling Pushup on Knees, Normal Pushup (as seen), Decline Pushup, Plyometric "Clap" Pushup.

Poor Technique:

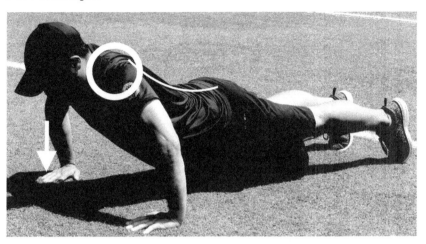

If you think this looks really bad, then wait until the next few illustrations! Hopefully you realize without explanation that I am way overarching the spine as shown by the curved white line. The white circle shows a shoulder shrug (commonly seen as a compensation for upper-body weakness) and the white arrow shows the elbow flaring out to a near 90-degree angle. As silly as this may look, I have seen too many athletes (yes, athletes!) look pretty similar to this overacting attempt of mine.

Staggered Stance Bent Over Unilateral Row

Upper Body: Unilateral Movement Patterns

Pull

Illustration shows proper pull through around ¾ the full range of motion with good alignment.

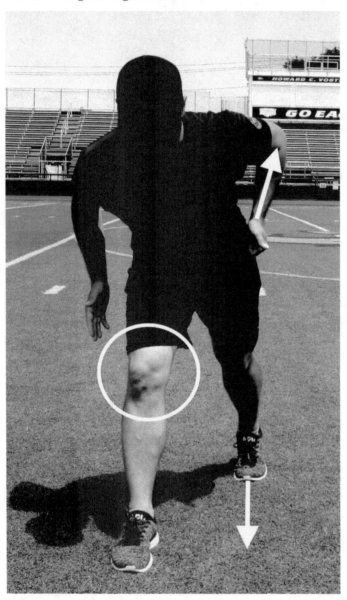

A staggered stance single-arm pulling movement is a great way to challenge your overall stability while performing this fundamental movement pattern. The staggered position is a good position to train and rehab with as it provides a slight level of inherent instability that requires higher internal stabilization demands of the body, particularly the core! The white circle shows good alignment of the front knee (don't forget about the lower half of the body when working on the upper body). The lower white arrow shows the foot positioned well straight ahead and the upper white arrow shows my elbow about a 30-45 degree angle away from my side. Note that conventionally we have been taught not to bring the elbow or upper arm behind the side of our body, which, besides some clinical applications based on individual needs, is outdated thinking. We utilize our shoulder both in front of (flexion) and behind (extension) our body so we should load it in both, however, do keep in mind: We have significantly more shoulder flexion (normally from 165-180 degrees) then shoulder extension (normally between 50-70 degrees).

Variations of this movement (from easier to challenging): Prone (laying on stomach) row off side of table or bed, seated single arm mid row, seated high to low single arm row, standing single arm mid row, standing high to low single arm row, staggered stance single arm mid row, staggered stance bent over single arm row (as seen), single arm overhead pull down.

Poor Technique:

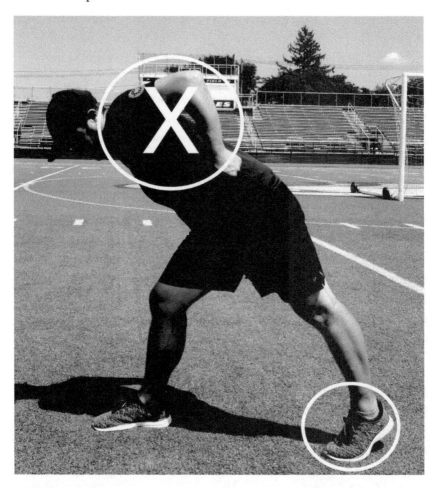

I hope I am meeting your expectations in showing sloppy technique!
Although there exist applications where lifting the heel is fine, lifting
the back foot is a common mistake made in the staggered position.
The really sloppy big white circle with X marking the spot is displaying
another common compensatory movement where the individual lacks
a vertical line of pull with the lower arm. A good way to self-audit your
pull is to check if your forearm is perpendicular to whatever resistance
is being pulled. So if it is a dumbbell then the line of pull is straight
down to the ground, and if it is a band anchored in front of you the
angle will be slightly different.

Staggered Stance Unilateral Push (Landmine Press)

Upper Body: Unilateral Movement Patterns

Push

Illustration shows proper push through the full range of motion with good alignment.

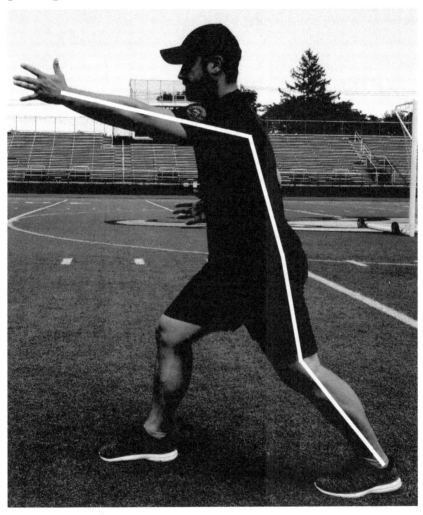

You might be looking at this wondering whether I am showing you a strange self-defense pose or a movement pattern. This movement is a favorite of mine as it is very relevant to overhead athletes and baseball players that are looking for safe and effective ways to train the upper body into pushing movements. Baseball players spend a ton of time throwing so there has been controversy related to loading pushing-based movements.

This movement shows a staggered stance single-arm press that you may have seen elsewhere known as a Landmine Press with a barbell slanted on an angle with one side gripped in the pushing hand. What you see is what you get with the white lines: Good alignment! Of importance to note is the finish for this movement. When we push as far as we feel our arm allows, we usually have additional movement that comes from our shoulder blades. The movement is similar to the end exaggeration of a straight punch, or as some might be familiar with the plus portion of a pushup or any press. This is important as we get plenty of shoulder range of motion from our ball and socket (glenohumeral) joint as well as our shoulder blade (scapulothoracic joint).

Variations of this movement (from easier to challenging): Supine (laying on back) light dumbbell press, Half-kneeling Single-Arm Horizontal Press, Single-Arm Incline Bench Press, Staggered Stance Landmine Press (as seen), Single-Arm Seated Overhead Press, Single-Arm Standing Overhead Press, Single-Arm Bottoms Up Kettlebell press

Poor Technique:

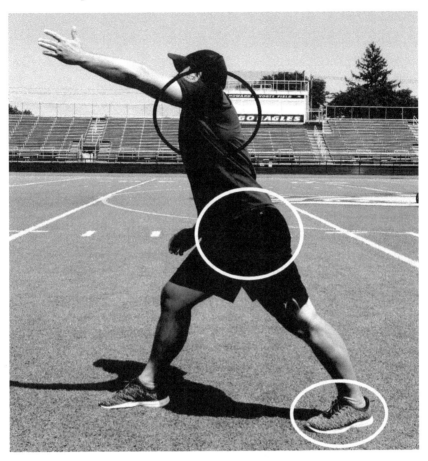

Is this the sloppiest display yet, or does it just look like another random pose? Before you read on, challenge yourself to find the compensatory patterns, *hint* *hint* it's in the circles!

The back foot is turned out and the middle circle shows the left hip opening and off-balance, and the top circle shows a shrug of the shoulder and a sidebending away from the pushing side.

Unilateral Farmer's Carry

Loaded Carry

Illustration shows proper unilateral loaded carry with a dumbbell.

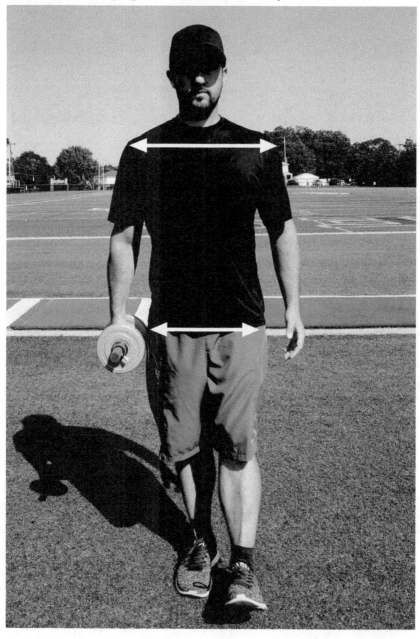

A loaded carry is an integral loaded movement to be included in your workout regimen and is the last of the nine fundamental movement patterns that I believe should constitute any solid performance-oriented strength training program. The goal with these nine forms of exercise is to build resilience through functional patterns of movement. A loaded carry has many benefits including:

◆ Incorporates the lower and upper half into an exercise simultaneously
◆ Challenges the body's overall postural stability, hips, and core
◆ Can work to increase overall workload capacity
◆ Functional carry over to normal tasks
◆ Trains grip strength which is correlated to overall shoulder muscle activation
◆ Vast ways to regress and progress the exercise

A good starting point for those that might not have performed this movement prior is to aim for sets of 30-45 second bouts of carrying weight anywhere from 30-40% of your body weight in one hand. Work up to 60 second + bout sets as your workload capacity increases with time. Note in the picture above how my hips are maintaining an even height during the walk, while my shoulders are also even and in a relaxed position.

Variations of this movement (from easier to challenging, assuming overall weight is the same): Trap Bar Carry, Suitcase Farmer's Carry (bilateral), Bilateral Rack Position Farmer's Carry with Kettlebell, Unilateral Rack position Farmer's Carry with Kettlebell, Bilateral Waiter's Position Farmers Carry, Unilateral Waiter's Position Farmer's Carry, Unilateral Overhead Farmer's Carry, Unilateral Bottoms Up Kettlebell Farmer's Carry.

Poor Technique:

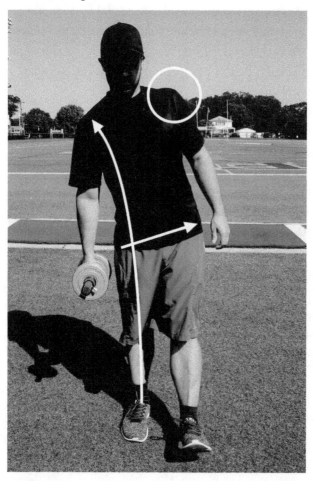

Note a few commonly seen compensatory patterns including the long white arrow showing a side-bending towards the side with the weight, uneven hip height, and a shrugged left shoulder. As you have learned in all of these nine fundamental movements, you should control your body by finding a neutral alignment throughout all major joints of the body.

Good job! You just graduated from Fundamental Movement Patterns 101. But instead of a certificate or course credit, you get the gift of the knowledge to begin to build your own individualized workout program.

4. Elastic Power

I believe that you are probably very interested in becoming as powerful as possible in your given activity. Whether you are a baseball or softball player looking to hit the ball further or throw harder, or a soccer player looking to improve your leg power, or any other type of performer looking to jump higher and run faster, regaining your power might be the sexiest part of going from injured to elite. The scientific definition of *power* is basically the ability to perform a certain amount of work within a certain amount of time. Putting it in the form of a math equation, you would include the variables of mass, acceleration, and time. Think of power as the motion that results from application of force in a given amount of time, or the change in work with respect to time. For the math geeks out there that are smarter than me, the equation for power is expressed as Power=Work/Time (P=W/T). Jumping slightly ahead to speed, since they are so commonly and incorrectly used interchangeably, the equation for speed is Speed=Distance/Time (S=D/T). The difference in these equations is that one refers to work while the other involves distance. Power is influenced by the amount of work performed, whereas speed is simply a measure of change in distance over time.

Using an example such as the speed of a bat swing in baseball (bat speed), think of what is being measured; the time that it takes for the bat to move a certain distance will give you bat speed, which is why it is expressed as miles per hour, or revolutions per minute. Interestingly, in baseball we refer to the ability to swing the bat hard and hit the ball far as power and not speed, yet we usually refer to bat speed, and exit velocity of the ball off the bat as measures of hitting *power*. The issue is that this does not account for the work being performed during a swing.

Stay with me here, as this will really move your understanding of performance beyond even many performance professionals. When you swing a bat there are many variables that can directly impact the power of that swing, such as the resistance of the air and the velocity of the ball coming towards the batter. Bat speed will not be directly affected by these factors since it does not measure the internal elements of the individual rather measuring the external aspect of movement (distance over time). The power of a swing will be directly impacted by these factors since the individual will have to perform more work to overcome these variables.

Amidst this most exciting section that probably took you back to unpleasant experiences sitting through dry science lectures (perhaps I am speaking for myself), the take-home point is this: power measures internal forces whereas speed measures external quantities (time and distance) of a body serving as a point of reference. What does this mean? Well, take into consideration that the distance covered in any given amount of time will most certainly require a certain level of power! As a matter of fact, the more power you express the greater the distance that can be covered. Sure, the speed of a ball off a bat, or out of the hand is great to know, and can sound impressive, but the power expressed by the body which is holding those objects is really at the root of what is allowing for this speed of movement in a given direction (velocity). And bringing it home, this is the reason why the bigger athletes swinging objects, tend to hit and throw them "harder" allowing for more work to be performed as you will soon learn.

Without understanding the importance of power first, measuring the speed of a moving body (even your own) does not give you "powerful" data on its own. This is why we are covering power before discussing speed. In order to develop speed, we must train our ability to be explosive and have ways to actually measure power.

One last concept to understand related to power is *elasticity*. Without getting any more technical, *elastic energy* can be thought of as that which is stored in a rubber band when it is stretched. Our tendons (the tissue that connects our muscles to bones) undergo a massive stretch prior to explosive movements. The energy that is stored during the loading phase of a movement can also be used during the explosive part of the movement and assist with the shortening of muscles. We call this process the stretch-shortening cycle. This is why performance coaches cue athletes to explode without pausing at the bottom portion of a movement as doing so can dissipate stored elastic energy.

Plyometric-based exercises such as medicine ball throws, or box jumps also utilize this concept of the stretch-shortening cycle. Another way to think of this is a coil compressing and then rapidly expanding with the stored energy, although instead of passively, it is happening actively during the muscle contractions while the muscle is both lengthening (stretching) and shortening.

So putting it together, to be powerful is the ability to perform work or move quickly with the application of internal forces. This leaves power training wide open to many different methods with the amount of work performed as the single most important element to power training. The most unique element of power especially from speed is force. Now, take a nice reset breath as we bring in the physics!

The equation for *work* is work=force×distance (w=f•d), therefore we must understand force to train power, and force=mass×acceleration (f=m•a). acceleration=change in velocity/change in time. Now we see that velocity (speed in a given direction) is just one part of power. So the most complicated variable to figure out during power movements is really force since it factors in acceleration, which is probably the most difficult number to quickly assess during any given exercise.

The bottom line is this; if you want to train power then you better have a way to measure it, otherwise this much more complicated concept will not be effectively harnessed in your program. If I have done nothing else than confuse or bore you, at least take the point that power is very often misrepresented and made difficult to understand. This is the reason why performing any powerful movement or exercise will not always translate to better performance. Of course, power is very necessary, but skill still has way more carryover as it pertains to performance. Objectively, you will need to work on both. The reason why skill is not one of the seven tools of performance is because skill is really a combination of all of them. Power alone will not lead to increased performance, but improving all areas of performance will cumulatively positively influence skill. However, skill alone does not lead to performance since there are many external variables when it comes to sports, including simple chance, or luck, that also influences overall performance.

Now getting back to power and recapping what you have just learned: The most difficult number to quantify will be force (mass * acceleration), since work=force×distance, and distance is much easier to figure out. If you are just putting more weight onto a barbell or jumping onto a higher box, you are still not necessarily factoring in acceleration. Remember, the weight might be increasing, but if the acceleration is not, then this will not fully translate to developing power. Power development requires forceful movements which are quickly performed, whereas speed does not factor in anything other than distance and time.

My challenge for you is to find a way to measure the acceleration of your power development activity. For example, an Olympic weightlifter's job is to lift as much weight as possible. However, just stacking weights onto the bar does not necessarily give them feedback about the bar path acceleration during the movement. Knowing the bar path acceleration can give actionable information related to their output of power. In this case, measuring bar speed does not require investing thousands of dollars into any fancy equipment (though there are devices out there like Bar Sensei that do measure bar speed). A good old-fashioned stopwatch or video recording can give you some of that basic information just as well. The goal should be to perform more work— fully executing the intended movement in the minimal amount of time. Take note, it is skill that will usually translate this power into an effective way towards your performance-related goals.

While writing this chapter, I consulted Jonathan Larson, my former strength and conditioning colleague with the St. Louis Cardinals, to get his opinion on training for power. During our time with the Cardinals, to lighten the mood for the players, we would introduce ourselves as the guy who breaks the athletes (Jonathan), and the guy who fixes them (me). When I asked him his thoughts on what to share with readers about power, he made a very strong point, he stated: "...the intent to develop power is more important than demonstrating and displaying power." His point was essentially that any exercise that appears to be powerful or explosive is not necessarily one that best helps develop your power.

In order to make sure that you are working on power, ask yourself if you are breaking down the exercise in a specific-enough way that you can do it at a certain percentage of your maximum ability and also quantify the acceleration of the movement. *Accommodating resistance* is a variable amount of resistance/load throughout the range of motion of a particular exercise or movement which can serve as a great way for individuals to train their ability to generate power. An example of accommodating resistance is a band-resisted speed squat which allows for effective acceleration. As the individual reaches towards the top of the squat there is greater tension on the band demanding increased force output. Another example is utilizing chains on a barbell during a bench press which decreases the load towards the bottom of the movement as the chains hit the ground and no longer provide resistance until reaching the top of the movement. Manipulating this amount of load at the negative phase of the movement allows for greater acceleration early on in the movement, and hence a greater ability to develop power.

Another form of popular power training in the world of strength and conditioning is The Conjugate Method. This type of training was popularized under the Westside training philosophy created by Louise Simmons who was influenced by his research into training programs of the former Soviet Union. This method programs in heavy days of training a specific movement or exercise, followed by "dynamic" days where you are taking on significantly less than a maximal external load while emphasizing speed of movement and higher amounts of volume or repetitions. This combines the importance of both acceleration and force on different days, both of which contribute to power development. My colleague, Jonathan Larson, has successfully utilized these principles with many high-performing athletes over the years, achieving great results.

The Conjugate Method allows the individual to effectively increase their overall workload in a manner that makes sense. As we learned in our physics lesson earlier, $force = mass \times acceleration$, therefore these dynamic days are integral parts of increasing overall force output and, since $work = force \times distance$, effectively training power. Yet, if you were to only train a movement slowly within a specific amount of range of motion (the distance), then though you are performing some level of work, you are not accounting for acceleration. On the other hand, if you were only training quickly with the thought of acceleration, then you would not be accounting for mass in order to increase your overall workload. Combining these two principles allows you to train power more completely.

Again, during dynamic days of training you will need some way of measuring acceleration, whether it is simply your rate of perceived exertion as discussed earlier, a simple stopwatch, video, or fancier equipment, including sensors. Work on power in a way that is specific to your activity instead of simply simulating movements of your activity at a high rate of speed. If you are a runner this doesn't only mean training power by simply running with a parachute, or sprinting uphill. Training power might mean working on single leg plyometric work in succession or of other methods that might allow for better measuring and quantifying.

I expect that you are now leaps and bounds ahead of your previous understanding of power and sports performance and you didn't even need to go formally study exercise physiology (though formal study doesn't hurt). All we needed instead was to look at a few basic physics equations. If you are a performance professional, maybe even you were reminded of a few oft-forgotten principles! Before concluding this section, here are some examples of how performance professionals measure power output:

- Power Output in Watts Displayed on Keiser's Pneumatic Resistance System:
    - Similar to a cable-and-pulley based system that you may find in a gym setting but digital so that it can give you feedback in terms of the level of power output that is generated during any given movement. This device is heavily used in the sports performance world.
- Vertical Jump Testing
    - This device estimates your vertical jump height (correlated to power output) based off of your foot

contact time interval between jumping off the mat and landing back onto the mat. Those that follow the NFL Combine may be familiar with the vertical jump test that uses a pole and elevated arms which laterally protrude off of the pole that the athlete attempts to hit with their hand. This tells their jump height. The jump mat system utilizes a digital approach to the same idea.

◆ Hop Testing (Lower Body Power)
   ○ Hop testing can consist of a battery of different hopping variations such as the single leg triple hop test, single leg hop for distance, crossover hop for distance, broad jump for distance, and timed hop test. The values are used as a functional indicator of lower extremity power and strength as well as overall symmetry. This testing is commonly done as part of the return-to-sport process following a knee surgery such as an Anterior Cruciate Ligament (ACL) reconstruction.

◆ Med Ball Throw Testing (Upper Body Power)
   ○ Just as hop testing aims to measure lower extremity power, the medicine ball throw test can indicate overall upper body power output. Some protocols include measuring the throwing distance of a chest pass using a weighted medicine ball, whereas others include sensors in the ball which can measure power output.

Remember that when you are developing power after injury, if you missed any necessary previous steps, this is where you will experience the law of diminishing returns; skipping ahead into an activity without completing the steps needed before starting to train power (and returning that power back to previous baseline levels) will only hinder the recovery process; if a weak link in the chain still exists, then you'll need to return to the missing step in order to effectively develop your power. An example is power output in a lower extremity after knee surgery. Our quadricep muscle is the most forceful muscle that crosses our knee joint. If you miss integral steps such as normalizing the function of the quadricep muscle when simply walking, then moving forward you will likely not activate the quadricep muscle fully, instead relying on other muscle groups that you're not intending to primarily train. Earlier in this chapter when discussing quality of movement, you learned that loading a poor movement pattern just enhances the impairment, and the same holds here with developing power — If you jump ahead without hitting the foundational elements of movement, you will just accentuate poor form related to the issue that you'd glossed over.

Do not make the mistake of ignorantly pushing ahead only to discover in hindsight that you'd missed fundamental steps. By that time, it may be too late and your whole recovery plan will be thrown into chaos. Don't be afraid of getting your team members involved to check that you are being deliberate in the steps you're taking. With the Injured to Elite process, it is more important to be thorough than quick.

5. Speed

Now that we have gotten the more confusing tool of power out of the way, it should be easier to understand speed. Speed is distance covered over a period of time (speed=distance/time). Keep in mind that speed differs from acceleration since acceleration is the change in speed over a specific change in time, and that the measure of speed has no specific direction or to use the more technical term, vector. Basically, speed is a scalar quantity which does not factor in the direction of an object, whereas velocity does factor in direction of movement, known as the vector of the object.

When we refer to speed in sports performance, we are generally referring to the measure of quickness over a specific amount of distance, such as the amount of time it takes to run the 40-yard dash. If we were talking golf, we might be referring to the club head speed, or in boxing, a fighter's ability to move a certain distance away from their opponent in the shortest amount of time to avoid a punch.

Almost every elite performer will need some type of speed,

whether it is the ability to climb a mountain quicker, or run down a field in less time. Therefore, what are some general guidelines you can follow to develop speed? Remember, always keep your training as relevant as possible to your specific activity — train speed-specific activities that can also carry over to your greater goals.

Speed Concept #1: Speed is easy to measure, but difficult to manipulate.

Compared with power, work, and acceleration, it's pretty easy to measure speed. Most of us have calculated the numbers needed to figure out speed — the finishing time and distance covered — without even thinking about it. Part of the reason for this is that relatively few controllable variables exist out there that affect speed. This makes it easier to track but difficult to manipulate, since all you can really change is your effort level and distance to cover. The result is that training speed takes a more direct, long-term approach. Don't expect to significantly increase your speed in just a few short weeks. Focusing on the other tools of performance will likely help give you a good baseline level of speed first.

Speed Concept #2: Aim to improve 2.5-5% closer to your goal each session.

Since there aren't many tweaks you can make to improve speed, the most straightforward approach to training speed is to use the same principle shared in the load management section of this book by figuring out an end goal related to speed and reverse-engineering your training plan to move towards that goal. In my experience, a realistic aim is to get 2.5-5% closer to your goal each session.

Let's say your goal is to run a 40-yard dash in 4.5 seconds, and your current baseline speed is 40 yards in five seconds. Now that we know your baseline and intended goal, we can make a plan to fill in the gap. Just as a successful business plan should have financial projections that are modest in nature, our aim should be realistic. So let's figure out how much time you'll need to get to your goal if you are able to improve by 2.5-5% during each session.

To start, you are looking to increase your time by half a second (.5), which is a very bold goal, but a convenient figure to use as an example. Bear with me as we get into some math here. As a side note, math was my least favorite subject in school, and yet here I am using it regularly in my profession! Anyway, if you are going to decrease your time by 2.5-5% of .5 seconds each session, you would first multiply .5 second by 2.5-5% to know exactly how much you need to improve each time (0.0125 to 0.025 of a second). You'll then divide .5 by this amount to determine approximately how many sessions you'll need to accomplish the goal (20-40 sessions). If you were to train and test your speed every single day, you would need a minimum of 3-7 weeks of training. However, you will likely need at least 1-3 day of recovery between sessions, so let's assume that you will complete 2-3 sessions per week as a top priority in your performance program. This would mean it would take at a minimum of seven weeks and maximum of twenty weeks overall, if you divide 20-40 training sessions by 2-3 sessions per week. On average, then, this will take around 3-4 months of training to get close to your very ambitious goal assuming everything goes very smoothly. In reality, you should add a few extra weeks to your estimate to account for unforeseen circumstances and "rainy days." 4 months is a reasonable amount of time here, allowing you to miss a few sessions in case of interruptions due to, to give a few examples: The common cold, bad weather, or a family emergency.

Generally, goals such as increasing speed should be off-season priorities if you partake in a sport with any type of off-season. Even if you don't, you should be giving yourself at least around 6-8 weeks of an off-season every year in order to reset, reflect, and re-focus your efforts away from competitive activities, that is along with at least 2-4 weeks of near total rest. This brings us to our next speed concept.

Speed Concept #3: Your speed goal should not exceed the length of your "off-season."

This concept may come off as basic common sense, but it is still important to note. Ideally, your speed goal should be completed in less time than your off-season and if you have other goals for the off-season, then you need to account for those as well. This means that the example above would actually only work for an individual that has an off-season of at least 4-5 months, if we include the recommended 2-4 weeks of total rest in the off-season. That's why I should repeat that the goal of increasing a half-second on the 40-yard dash is a very aggressive goal to be completed in one off-season and was only used here for math purposes. If you do not have an off-season, then this concept still holds true for a less intense portion of your year.

The point is that you must set your goals within the framework of what is realistic within your yearly schedule. You can certainly break up the goal throughout different phases of the year but remember that whenever you are working towards such an ambitious goal, you will need to make full use of the other tools of performance, especially since you will also be focusing some of your efforts on recovery, in addition to other elements of training. Even without injury, increasing speed takes enough work that it becomes difficult to compete at your best while working on increasing your overall speed performance, so set your priorities wisely.

Speed Concept #4: Use an appropriate activity-specific measure for speed.

If you are not engaging in a sport or activity that requires running, then don't blindly begin a sprinting speed program just to feel like you are training effectively as an athlete. Speed can mean a lot of things for different sports and, as previously mentioned, has a lot of crossover into power. Whether you are a boxer looking to improve the speed of your movements to better your defense, or a dancer looking to increase the rate of your spinning movements, you must figure out a way to objectively measure speed as related to that activity. Without

195

this measure, none of what I've written above will matter since you won't be able to tell when you've achieved your goal in the context of your needs.

6. Cognitive-Perceptual Performance

Brain training, mental performance, mind/body training, and neurofeedback are just some of the many terms that you might be familiar with related to cognitive-perceptual performance (CPP). For many of you, including performance professionals who might be reading this, CPP will be a new idea, since it has only recently begun to gain a following.

If we break down this term, we see that cognitive refers to mental processing and perceptual refers to our conscious recognition and interpretation of sensory information. Cognitive-perceptual performance can be defined as the level of ability we have to integrate information given to us from our senses in order to make decisions that are related to our performance. In my experience over the past several years, this is the area which performance teams within the world of professional and collegiate athletics are devoting more and more time and money towards building. In fact, it is no longer acceptable for organizations to put an athlete on a strength and conditioning workout program without also considering CPP. The same should hold for you since you've got some time away from competition while healing.

Optimizing your cognitive-perceptual abilities can have a tremendous impact on your performance in both daily life and sport. I was exposed to an advanced form of this training while working at ADI Rehab in Los Angeles. Sean Hampton, partially owns and operates Neurovision Consulting (www.neurovision-med.com), a company that assesses and trains cognitive-perceptual capability. The baseball players that I sent over to Neurovision would make statements like "... the ball now seems like it is slowing down!" when describing how it felt hitting after performing several weeks of training. The system would objectively break down and assess specific elements of the individual's cognitive-perceptual performance including depth perception, peripheral depth perception, executive functioning (ability to quickly make decisions based on information), mental skills acquisition, and motion perception. The baseline assessment entails specific tracking of eye movements under certain circumstances, prior to training. Neurovision then utilizes a device called the neuro-tracker which shows various 3-dimensional balls on a screen that race around while the individual tracks and recalls them through their movement on the screen while wearing 3D glasses.

The training element of Neurovision differs from many of the other systems out there, such as those that require wearing strobe-like glasses for a technique called optical occlusion training. Optical occlusion training, another form of cognitive-perceptual performance training, partially obstructs your vision while requiring you to perform a certain task. Over my career, I have had the opportunity to utilize this technique as well.

Neurovision is unique among other advertised "brain training" devices in that it actually first measures baseline levels of cognitive-perceptual performance metrics related to vision. Other systems out there, such as optical occlusion training, do not measure those specific elements, nor do they intentionally manipulate them using guided protocols like the Neurovision system does. Closing your eyes during an exercise is just about as effective as optical occlusion training in terms of CPP; it is related more to our body awareness (*proprioception*) abilities rather than directly and specifically targeting our central processing abilities. For best results, these systems should include a formal assessment process, as well as a training program with specific protocols that focus on correcting the deficiencies found using that assessment.

Another example of a growing CPP training tool is the FITLIGHT Trainer, which incorporates LED light sensors that turn specific colors indicating a specific task to be performed. The user is then required to tap the light with whatever movement is indicated by the color of the light to activate the rest of the training sequence. This system is somewhat similar to the Bop It toy you might remember from childhood. A benefit to this training system is the ability for users to creatively design their own reaction training protocols, allowing for some specificity in their routine. One of the drawbacks is that the device will not always be able to accurately detect if a correct task was performed. For example, if a user decides to create a protocol that includes tapping one of the strategically placed light sensors with only their left hand, it will not be able to sense this detail since it can only respond to general contact or proximity. While working with Neurovision colleagues, I spent time experimenting with the FITLIGHT system in order to figure out novel ways to increase mental processing during use by adding complexity to exercises and by asking the athlete to complete additional tasks while reacting to the device. After experimenting, I felt that it certainly added an engaging dynamic element to conventional exercises, but I struggled with the idea that there is very limited ability to perform any level of baseline testing or the ability to train specific elements of cognitive perceptual performance. If you are after improving reaction time, then it could potentially be effective, but know that the FITLIGHT is not a jack-of-all-trades training device for the many other elements of CPP.

In almost all cases, this area of performance requires a well-qualified technician who understands how to test and train different elements of CPP. What are some ways you can work on this at home right now, even if you don't happen to have your own mental skills and performance coach? The most important first step is to define what you are looking to improve. Is it your focus on a specific task or ability to lock-in? Are you looking to react quicker physically to something by making faster decisions? Do you want to improve your ability to track some type of object? Are you dealing with some level of performance anxiety or fear that is influencing your mental performance? Perhaps you want to improve your ability to persevere mentally in stressful situations. Once you identify what you intend to address, then you can decide how to improve it.

The overarching concept of cognitive-perceptual performance of the Injured to Elite Method is to define what element of mental performance or CPP that you are looking to address instead of expecting any brain training program to carry over in ways that you desire. Below are several ways to improve CPP for some of the most commonly desired areas:

Performance Anxiety and Fear

For the most part, tools to deal with performance anxiety and fear have been detailed in chapter five. That being said, in my experience working with hundreds of elite athletes after injury, performance anxiety and fear are some of the most prevalent obstacles in the way of their journey towards unlimited performance, so I feel it is worthwhile to include a little more on overcoming these obstacles.

When you find yourself in a state of anxiety or fear you often look for elements outside of yourselves that can save you from the stressor, whether that is a brace, pill, or another person. In reality, the answer frequently lies within you. Instead of resisting the physical, emotional, and mental symptoms of fear and anxiety associated with your injury and performance, it is more helpful to directly face it head on. Utilizing the following steps, which don't require anything outside of your own resources, can come to your rescue. They will get easier each time you flex this new muscle of yours, so don't be discouraged if it feels out-of-reach at first.

1. Imagine being one with whatever source is causing fear and anxiety. If it is, for example, fear of reinjuring a specific body part and the physical pain associated with that, go a bit deeper into that feeling for 5-10 seconds.
2. Imagine that feeling gently fading away as you become one with this obstacle.
3. Focus on a thought of gratitude that relates to your recovery. This can be a grateful thought for something that has served you well through this seemingly difficult time. It can also be a thought of gratitude for something that simply brings you good feelings, like still being able to work towards your goals despite your injury. Perhaps it is simply being grateful for your own ability to persevere!
4. Perform the reset breath as instructed in chapter five, and go boldly forward with the task at hand.

It may have felt like anxiety and fear had an overwhelming hold on you up until this point but through your strength of intention, you can get over them, and actually let them fuel you. Indeed, you will learn how a higher sense of purpose can intensify your perseverance through these moments in the coming chapters. Before moving on, I want to tell you that if your anxiety or fear become overwhelming, there is no shame in seeking help. The Association for Applied Sports Psychology is an incredible resource for getting connected with someone locally and in-person. Just go to their website at www.appliedsportspsych. org/resources/resources-for-athletes. There you will find a wealth of information for athletes looking to overcome these challenges.

Reaction Timing and Executive Decision-Making

This refers to the ability to quickly make a decision like figuring out where to throw a ball or, metaphorically speaking, training when to "pull the trigger" when a lightning-quick decision has to be made. To train this quality, one option is the FITLIGHT system mentioned earlier. It does have a bit of a learning curve to operate therefore might not be the best for those looking to train on their own, not to mention its high price. At the time of writing, a great free option is the mobile app SwitchedOn Training, with its slogan: "Perceive. Decide. React Faster." The application allows the user to perform drills created by performance experts to train both reaction time and quick decision-making. This device is much more cost effective and practical than many of the other sports performance tech toys in this category, however it is still relatively new as far as its development goes. Whether it is truly effective is not completely clear from research, but it does seem to show promise. Moreover, this system embodies the Injured to Elite tenant of taking ownership of the healing process.

Focus and Attention

Neurofeedback is a system which non-invasively taps into your brain waves and works on optimizing them with sound frequency and visual stimulation. Research has shown that sound frequency has a direct impact on our brain waves. In the recovery section of this book we discussed how certain states have associated brain wave patterns, including sleep. Another example of using sound to heal is "sound baths." Goldsby et al (2017)[19] studied 62 individuals who underwent Tibetan sound meditation and found a decrease in post-meditation levels of physical pain in members of the study aged 40-59. The study also found decreased levels of tension, anger, fatigue, and depressed mood, especially in those trying the therapy for the first time. Though this study wasn't perfect (it lacked randomization, for example, and had a relatively small sample size), it was a positive beginning for an area lacking previous research. Despite a lack of research, sound baths have become quite popular in the alternative medicine community. A more straightforward example is studying with classical music playing, which, some say, improves focus.

Through my working relationship and friendship with Major League pitcher, Ryan Sherriff, I was introduced to a specific neurofeedback device that he used in Culver City, California, called BrainKanix (www.brainkanix.com). After watching Ryan work with the device and tell me about his positive experience with it, I gave it a shot myself. Painless electrodes that are attached to a helmet-like device are placed on your head along with wearing headphones while you sit and watch a monitor which displays transforming multi-colored shapes. The premise is that as your brain waves are evaluated by the device, it uses sound and visual stimulation in order to optimize them. I did not perform enough treatment sessions to feel an effect, but there is evidence that it works. It is even being used in several rehab centers to change the brain waves of those suffering from addiction. My favorite feature of this device is that the user does not really need to do much

19   Goldsby, T. L., Goldsby, M. E., McWalters, M., & Mills, P. J. (2017). Effects of Singing Bowl Sound Meditation on Mood, Tension, and Well-being: An Observational Study. *Journal of Evidence-Based Complementary & Alternative Medicine*, 22(3), 401–406. https://doi.org/10.1177/2156587216668109

other than sit still, which can feel quite relaxing. The device utilizes an alpha-theta training protocol which rewards the alpha and theta brain waves of the individual. Our alpha and theta brain waves are part of our sleep/wake cycle and specifically the more "in-between" states of twilight. The idea behind this training protocol is that it may help resolve inner conflicts that might be causing stress and anxiety, by bringing these subconscious thoughts to the surface.

Our brain has electrical activity just like the rest of our body, however since we think of our brain as the control center of our body, logically the brain has its own complex electrical signaling system. This system can be detected, monitored, and tracked by the use of an electroencephalogram (EEG). Similar to how an EKG is performed to check our cardiac electrical activity, the same can be done for our brain. What the research has found is that our brain has specific wave states of electrical activity that can be associated with different states of arousal and cognitive functioning. Neurofeedback is a means in which an external system can provide our brain with feedback to encourage specific brain waves to become more prevalent.

BrainKanix is one system which does this by providing auditory and visual stimulation that serves as feedback based on the electrical activity detected by the system. First, the individual performs a test where the system is able to better understand that individual's brain activity during a specific task. When the actual training starts, the individual watches a screen while wearing the headset which trains these specific brain waves by rewarding them to become more prevalent. You can think about our brain as having a less evolved way of self-regulating based off of its brain waves. Have you ever wondered why you can't stay focused even though you've set a goal to get a task completed on a particular day? These answers may lie within our brain waves, and our brain's ability to self-monitor and regulate them to fit our specific goals and intentions.

So what does the research say about all of this? Well, systems such as BrainKanix that use neurofeedback devices can work on training specific brain waves such as our alpha and theta waves known as an "alpha/theta protocol." These brain waves are our states of arousal in-between highly alert and deeper states of sleep. The studies on neurofeedback and alpha/theta training, which show that neurofeedback has the ability to improve focus and attention, are numerous and outlined in a review paper titled "EEG-neurofeedback for optimising performance. I: A review of cognitive and affective outcome in healthy participants" published in 2013 in the *Journal of Neuroscience and Biobehavioral Reviews*[20].

Improving your focus and attention will require that you develop new habits and get rid of old ones that haven't worked out well for you. Chapter 5, "Rehabbing Your Mind," taught you how to kickstart your journey towards building good habits with tools like meditation, journaling, and conscious breathing techniques. Just like you learned the importance of being present in order to take physiological control of your breathing, the power of being present can also help you capture your mind. If I have done my job well, you have learned that recovery requires being present with both your mind and body! It will take practice to break habits in your routine and improve your consistency — it's not easy. If you've put in the effort but you feel like you can't seem to make any more improvements, it is at that point when you might consider working one-on-one with a professional.

Visual Performance

If you don't have access to a company like Neurovision, there are other visual performance systems out there including Sports Vision EyeQ by RightEye and the Nike Sparq Sensory Station. These systems might be less practical for those who do not belong to a large sports organization who can purchase these big-ticket items, but stay on the lookout as these forms of training will eventually become more readily affordable and available to home users. In the meantime, I recommend consulting with your local eye specialist to see what might be available in your area when it comes to visual performance training.

Vision is extremely important to our performance so you

20   Gruzelier, John. (2013). EEG-neurofeedback for optimising performance. I: A review of cognitive and affective outcome in healthy participants. *Neuroscience and biobehavioral reviews*. 44. 10.1016/j.neubior-ev.2013.09.015.

should, at the very least, be seeing your eye doctor regularly. In fact, some professional sports teams are even using a visual assessment as a way of screening potential players. Going even further, it's safe to say that the days of just prescribing a pair of glasses or contact lenses are behind us, especially for high-performing athletes; the growth of visual performance training and procedures like LASIK and LASEK eye surgery have raised the bar when it comes to vision. All-star baseball player Ted Williams, one of the greatest hitters of all time, had a catch phrase: "See the ball, hit the ball." So do your best to work to make sure you can see what it is you are intending to do.

7. Support

Last, but not least, is support. This refers to both your ability to support yourself as well as the ability and desire of others in your life to offer you support. This topic has been gaining prominence in the field over time, in fact, the American Physical Therapy Association has been encouraging the profession to pay closer attention to what they call *psychosocial* factors, which can have a major influence on patient outcomes. Lots of factors are involved in your capacity to cope with the many bumps in the road including your grit score, overall self-confidence, presence of family/close friends, the general quality of your relationships, and the quality of your performance team. All of those are important, but having a high level of self-confidence, high grit score, and a top team serve you especially well.

Our level of confidence is ever-changing; sometimes we're flying high and sometimes we're down on ourselves. The latter can be most true when we are physically wounded. The big question is: How do you build up that confidence to overcome fear of re-injury, and lack of ability to perform? The entire journey from injured to elite is full of opportunities to build up your confidence. As a matter of fact, being full of confidence right after an injury isn't always ideal. As high-striving humans, it is easy for us to overshoot our goals too soon during these times if we rush into activities with a false sense of our abilities, so a dip in confidence actually serves as a self-protective mechanism. I've mentioned it before and I'll mention it again: Don't rush — confidence should be a state of knowing, not guessing.

Think back to the importance of "I am" affirmation statements from John Denney's Harmony Exercise (see chapter five). The affirmation statement you are looking to make here is "I am ready." Now, in order to be truly and authentically confident in making this statement, you must know what you're ready for. Use the principles of load management and momentum in order to dictate your progress — make intelligent plans, follow through with each step, and assess your progress frequently. Be confident in the process and you will regain confidence in your abilities. As John Denney professes: When you continue on this path, right action will occur, with you "...having trust and faith that all is working out in perfect order."

The Final Stretch

Appropriately enough, we are back to the spiritual side of our journey. Now it is time to enter the last section of *Injured to Elite* where we will use all that came before to bring together the different parts of your life and solidify the idea of total transformation.

You probably know that the hardest part of the physical journey is in gaining that last 5-10% of your performance. The law of diminishing returns tells us that over time, the same effort level, even if it's very high, will eventually gain less increase in output. It gets lonely when you are struggling to climb a mountain and are one of the only ones near the top. It's the same with this book, the advice from the previous chapters is simple to read, but a challenge to implement; many people don't have the passion and commitment to follow-through, so if you've gotten this far in both theory and practice, you should be incredibly proud of yourself. Just as with that last 5-10%, now is the time in the book to exude the maximum level of patience while continuing to dig as deep as you can in your mind, body, and spirit. While you may be the only one making the journey, you're not alone, remember to make use of your performance team, and all of the support system I discussed in the previous section. Let them help you now, so that you can all celebrate your victory.

Part III: Putting It All Together

"Are you going to win to be happy, or be happy to win?"

-John Denney

CHAPTER 8
USING YOUR MOMENTUM
TO FUEL OTHER AREAS OF
LIFE

We have reached the time to unify the mind, body, and spirit
in that much-needed transformation from injured to elite. We can
start off by saying that your spirit is the invisible and less tangible
part of your being that offers you the ability to tap into an infinite
source of energy. Your spirit ultimately connects your mind and
body to the outside world through a force which can not be fully
understood through science. I believe that it is this non-physical part
of existence which makes elite performance possible. The unthinkable
and incomprehensible physical abilities an individual possesses are
filled with this spiritual energy, which many believe connect with the
rest of the universe. The mind and body express one's spirit in a way
with which we can see, feel, and interact. When people experience
hardship, it is common for them to begin seeking the higher forces in
the universe. These higher forces can supply us with infinite energy to
express our true highest sense of self.

Olympic gold medalist, hall of famer, Rolling Stones performer,
and personal best record-setting champion are examples of how we may
visualize our highest sense of purpose. With a truly holistic approach,
in order to attain this peak level of performance, the mind, body, and
spirit must all come together. Sure, achieving this for ourselves sounds
great, but a higher sense of purpose must serve something greater than
just ourselves. This desire lives in our spirit, an insurmountable force
of goodness in the world. Those who are recovering from substance

abuse, coming out of abusive relationships, or overcoming a physical challenge, are in the exact position for a much-needed spiritual awakening. In a way, side-lined with an injury, there is no better time than right now for you to tap into your higher self.

Rehabbing your mindset will allow your brain to get out of the way and let your body recover at its best. Having the goal of becoming an elite athlete might be enough to drive your performance forward, but it is not enough to make a lifelong transformation that carries over into all aspects of your life. The Injured to Elite journey is taking you past just performance-oriented goals and towards a more fulfilled and purposeful life. Now that you've pressed the reset button, it is time to refocus your physical and mental goals, and just as importantly, to give attention to your sense of overall purpose.

A Sense of Purpose

How has this journey already changed you as an individual? What did you learn about yourself or others in your life during this physical and mental shift? What do you want to change in the future about yourself? What fears have you overcome which previously stood in your way? What is your *why statement* to achieve this elite level of physical performance? Is it to show others your capabilities? Are you doing this for someone other than yourself? Do you just want to earn a higher paycheck (though there are probably other, easier, ways), or is there another reason? Have you thought about what your contribution to the rest of the world is through your performance achievements? There is no question that you have grown through this process, but what is your level of contribution outside of yourself? The answers to these questions will fuel your entire life and all thanks to a challenge you faced head-on, your injury.

Many of the high-achieving professional athletes I've worked with do, in fact, make the effort to feed their spirit a whole lot more than many would expect. Sure, many of them buy fancy cars and houses, among many other things, to feel significant, but by performing at their best, they are also able to contribute to their communities.

Think of a curtain call, when an athlete comes back onto the field after an outstanding performance. This, in many ways, signifies their acknowledgement of the community they are serving (and vice versa). How about you, who is the community you are serving? What is your contribution? What is your higher sense of purpose? What does your performance mean beyond yourself? These questions shouldn't be so easy to answer right off the bat. Spend some time reflecting on the entire journey thus far — put the physical and mental goals aside for a moment and focus on your higher purpose. If it does not include contributing to the greater good, then continue reflecting on your journey until you find a way to see beyond yourself. If you are going to make this transformation towards living a more purposeful and fulfilled life, establishing a sense of higher purpose is one of the most necessary steps of the entire process. Having a higher purpose is like armor that protects you from being thrown off by setbacks, both physical and mental; interestingly, focusing on others makes *you* more resilient! Selfishly, you also tap into this sense of purpose (or your spirit) as a way of further increasing your performance in the moment.

For those that are struggling to figure out where to even begin in this spiritual search let me offer some assistance. Your higher self is ever-evolving, and the idea here is not to dictate a mission for the rest of your life, but rather to figure out what the driving force in your life is at present, and the *why* behind it. At this very moment what enduring mission are you on and why? If down the line you realize this whole pursuit was just to please someone else, there will come a time when living out someone else's purpose will no longer be enough; our spirit needs to be fed from the inside to be truly fulfilled.

Think beyond the physical outcome of your post-injury process, what will endure? Is it your ability to be a better friend, significant other, or parent? How can your journey inspire others who are in need of a transformation? Keep asking these questions and others that come to mind even if you aren't getting satisfying answers right away. I assure you, if you remain persistent, the answers will be revealed in time. Actually, the answers might be right under your nose, but you haven't spent enough focused effort to *see* them. One helpful strategy is to think in terms of gratitude — reminding yourself of all that you are thankful for is like a key that can unlock wisdom, and at least make you a little bit happier in the moment.

Seeking My Higher Self

If you need some inspiration then let me share a bit more of my own story on how I found my higher purpose in the midst of a career in professional sports. Ever since I can remember, my goal has been to be on the field with the New York Mets. Initially it was to be a player, but over time it evolved to becoming a performance specialist with the organization. Eventually, I was accepted into the Doctor of Physical Therapy program at NYU. While there, I asked one of my favorite professors —who I considered a mentor— about how I could break into professional sports as a physical therapist. He suggested that I network and develop relationships with sports agents and others representing professional athletes. But the details of how this would help still weren't totally clear to me at that time since physical therapists were still just getting a footing in professional sports. Even for my professor (through no fault of his own), my best path forward was not apparent. Historically, sports had been dominated by athletic trainers, so it was tough finding a physical therapist that could offer comprehensive advice. During my studies, I was able to complete some of the top sports physical therapy internships, and felt confident enough to accept my first job at a private sports outpatient PT clinic that saw a high volume of local high school, collegiate, and a few professional athletes, in Westchester, NY.

After getting a lot of repetition and volume seeing these patients, and starting a web-based PT application called Videohab. com to record your rehab exercises and track progress outside of the PT clinic, I decided I needed to further my sports medicine training. The decision of exactly how to do that was made at the Team Concepts Conference in Las Vegas, the biggest annual sports physical therapy conference. There, I crossed paths with Mike Reinold, one of my mentors and former Physical Therapist and Athletic Trainer for the

Boston Red Sox. Since I was searching for the next step, I asked Mike how to get myself into professional baseball (hopefully with the Mets). Mike recommended applying to the Hospital for Special Surgery (HSS) Sports Physical Therapy Residency, since HSS is the team medical provider and hospital for the New York Mets. This was the perfect advice for an ambitious physical therapist pursuing working towards my own high standards. Unsurprisingly, I took Mike Reinold's advice and applied to HSS.

Fast forward to my HSS Residency interview. I was sitting across from three of their senior staff members, or as I like to think of them, the HSS firing squad. When asked what my long-term goal was, I told them, "I want to be in the dugout after this residency," in other words, I wanted to be working for a Major League Baseball team. I will never forget the feedback they gave me. I was told, "...well maybe that won't happen in a year, but maybe it will happen in five years." Though that response was perfectly logical and appropriate, at the time I thought, "Uh-oh, I just messed up my chances of being selected as a Resident!" My fears were unnecessary. After I was chosen, Program Director John Cavanaugh told me that my vision for my career was actually one of the main reasons that they had chosen me to be the one annual resident.

Moreover, around six months after that interview, I became the first HSS Sports PT Resident to spend a day at Citi Field and go behind-the-scenes with the New York Mets medical training staff for a full game. If you've ever seen the movie *Rudy*, well, this was my Rudy moment! You see, you have to imagine being the son of a father who was an absolute die-hard fanatic of this team, and then you're being given the opportunity to work alongside them for a day. It was unbelievable! This is especially true for me because my father had passed away around eight years before, and since then all I'd wanted was a chance to make him proud. On that day, it felt like things were coming into place for the first time since the day he died, and I vowed to my family to uplift myself through the pain. That magical day remains my favorite memory in professional sports.

I worked hard and felt like I was on the way to my goal of breaking into professional baseball, but not in a million years would

I have guessed that just six short months later I would become the Medical and Rehab Coordinator for the St. Louis Cardinals. I mean, there's no way to predict such opportunities! I will never forget the moment I accepted the job because it was totally random. It was near the end of my time with HSS, and I was on a mountain in Lake Placid, NY, with the United States Olympic Committee helping out during a Bobsled and Skeleton World Cup event. At that time, I could not have guessed how my purpose and tangible goals would evolve over the next few years. My major goal went from simply working at the highest level in professional sports to..."Empower those facing physical challenges to transform their lives through an optimal state of body, mind, and spirit."

Getting to this deeper sense of my higher purpose only became possible after I went through a professional crisis (previously mentioned in chapter five) in which I questioned whether I wanted to work for a team or to serve athletes directly. My experience in professional sports showed me that, unfortunately, business came first, even in relation to the health of the athletes. This was something I struggled with since it didn't align with my personal and professional ethics of prioritizing patients/clients. This isn't to say that the teams I worked with didn't take good care of athletes, rather that, when it came down to it, their overall mission was different from mine; the purpose of a team is to win, whereas my purpose is to uplift and empower others to achieve greatness and fulfillment beyond just money and sports victories.

It was not a physical injury or specific emotional setback that I was dealing with, but in terms of my career it was the lowest point; after achieving my dream of working with a professional baseball team, I had to figure out what to do next. It was during that crises of confidence that I vowed to only aim for the highest sense of my own purpose and never settle for anything less. Though I had been blessed with financial and personal stability, and the work ethic and luck to have achieved my dream job at a relatively young age, I simply could not remain complacent — I had to get on the path towards my highest sense of purpose in this world. My wish is the same for each and every one of you readers.

The Story of Your Purpose

Going through Time Zero, you probably didn't think of it as an opportunity. Yet, what better time is there to truly seek or reexamine your sense of self and higher purpose?

It seems counterintuitive, but appreciating this gift — being grateful for the opportunity to have been injured — is, in itself, the fuel to become elite. Moreover, it is the key to achieving a fulfilled life regardless of the circumstances. Recall when earlier in this book I mentioned the pattern that I witnessed many professional-level athletes get into after injury. Rarely does an elite performer stay the same after injury; typically they either go on to greater success or their career fizzles out. One key difference is that the successful athletes keep the right mindset about injuries or setbacks, using them as slingshots to propel themselves forward.

One of the most important tenets of the Injured to Elite method is the call for you to decide how you will respond to your Time Zero. After all, it's your choice to make when you catch yourself descending into self-pity or sorrow. You can decide to give-in and let the pain and suffering take over, or you can decide to accept your feelings with gratitude for the gift you were given, and redirect that negative energy into fuel. Your sense of purpose is the backbone to it all.

Focusing on what you are grateful for in this journey, and how the process has transformed or reminded you of that sense of higher purpose is the jumping off-point. Rather than simply being results-oriented, your sense of achievement expands to encompass an idea of fulfillment in life that is holistic — not just sports, not just relationships, not just financial gain, but everything together aimed at a greater good that is meaningful to you; achieving your physical goals and helping your team win are not necessarily bad, but connecting your mind, body, and spirit at a time of obstacles far outweighs any temporary victories.

Instead of focusing on the results you are looking to achieve, spend some time living in the process. In the words of John Denney: "Are you going to win to be happy, or be happy to win?" The moments of conquest we strive for are usually fleeting and not long-lived anyway. There will always be new pains, new obstacles, new challenges to overcome, if there weren't, what would we call progress? If we get away from wishing those challenges away and start putting our intentions into continual right action, the results will speak for themselves; when you really look deep into your heart's desires and question what you are hoping to get out of this, you realize that you are seeking out an emotional state. Whether you want to feel powerful, excited, uplifted, or just plain happy, you are not required to wait for a specific achievement to experience these emotions. This is the same idea that you learned in the first section of this book, the concept of taking ownership of your mind and body. The empowered state of being in control of your emotions and physiological state is the force that will allow you to tap into your best self at any moment.

The irony here is that while the book is called *Injured to Elite*, once you're there, you will realize that achieving the level of elite becomes just an added bonus. The process of going from injured to elite is where the beauty lies — that is where the real transformation occurs. You must continue to focus on that process in all areas of your life.

CHAPTER 9
MAINTAINING HEALTH

"Long breath, long life; short breath short life"

Now that you have reached your physical goals and have found your higher sense of purpose through the Injured to Elite journey, how do you maintain your progress? Having your mind, body, and spirit all working together should be an unstoppable healing force against any physical injury, yet we humans have so many distractions and outside forces in our lives that make total focus difficult. Although as I mentioned earlier, a state of health is our natural condition, we do sometimes create obstacles to that state when we get off-track in life. How then do we get back to our natural state? All of the previous chapters have given you countless tools to help you stay on course, the challenge is to consistently incorporate them into your life. Early on in the process the quick results should entice you to stay with the program, however, once you attain some of your physical goals and heal from your injury, it becomes ever easier to neglect the strategies that got you there. Luckily, there is a specific plan to deal with this that is already ingrained within us.

Willpower is our ability to flip a switch that helps us overcome difficulty. It is what keeps us going and going even when things are tough. Willpower helps us make the right decisions to stay on the path towards high performance. There are no secrets or life hacks here. Engaging your willpower is just like back in chapter five when you created an anchor to flip the switch to control your emotional state upon encountering negative thought viruses — you use the same strategy when you feel like you are falling off-course.

If I were to add an eighth tool of performance in the Injured to Elite method, it would likely be willpower, the ability to recognize yourself slipping, and flip that switch. Think of your favorite athlete or performer and you will probably be able to identify moments when they have turned things up a notch, or seemingly flipped a switch that miraculously turned around a bad situation. There is no way to fully understand how willpower works other than that it must be a fully coordinated effort through the mind, body, and spirit.

The reset breath (also from chapter five) is another strategy to use when you are feeling lost or unfocused. Going back to that earlier chapter, the reset breath is a conscious breathing strategy. You take a time out with a nice deep diaphragmatic breath throughout your body, filling yourself with gratitude, and going forward. This simple activity has been with us since ancient times with many spiritual gurus professing: "Long breath, long life; short breath, short life."

Injury Prevention

A subject that I'm sure you've heard a lot about in the past and that you perhaps would have expected to see in this chapter is injury prevention. I have always felt strange about this idea of injury prevention, since if you logically buy in to the idea of completely preventing injury, you are likely also holding back on the field. There is an inherent risk when we push the limits of our performance, that's just a fact of high-level athletics. The fine line between pushing as hard as we can and too hard can have major implications, but the truth is that all we can do is mitigate or decrease risk factors — there's nothing that will keep you safe 100% of the time besides not playing. You have already worked on this yourself in the performance optimization chapter, where we discussed principles of self-assessing your weaknesses. Your performance team, led by you, should already be very well aware of the weak links in your chain, and you should have a routine that aims to stay on top of these weaknesses. The goal is not necessarily to change your weaknesses into strengths but rather to make sure to give them regular attention as you train.

You should plan specific, predetermined, times of the year when you re-evaluate your movement and progress. I advise performing a self-evaluation at least 1-2 times in-season and at least 1-2 times during the off-season. Think of this as something like a quarterly self-review. Below are a few questions you should answer and things to look for which you should note in your performance journal:

1. Have my basic movement patterns changed recently?
2. Have I lost range of motion or mobility in a specific joint?
3. Is my recovery on track?
4. Am I rating my effort level higher for activities that used to feel more effortless? If the answer is yes, this can be a warning sign for the need to better optimize load and recovery.
5. Has there been a steady improvement in my progress and overall workload? Ideally, the answer is yes most of the time, but there will be moments when it is totally normal not to see big changes here.

These quarterly reviews are also a good time to check-in with a performance professional in order to help you delve deeper into areas of your body that might need some fine-tuning. Remember, you don't need to have your hand held every day of the year, but it can be very helpful to check-in with some members of your team a few times throughout the year to reassess and note any changes.

No matter what you do there are eventually going to be viruses, colds, nagging aches and pains, small injuries, and even some significant injuries, but don't fear them. Remember how much you learned from your Time Zero event, and recognize that nothing can ever fully eject you from your transformation unless you allow it to. The Injured to Elite method is a lifelong process where you are always the director. Through the use of your willpower, you can emerge through any challenge and never fear losing yourself.

Fear

As Franklin D. Roosevelt stated in his 1933 inaugural address: "The only thing we have to fear is fear itself." If you find yourself in a state of fear, briefly review the mindset optimization chapter. It is the most important chapter in this book for everyone to regularly review (myself included). Now, think back to the reptilian brain, the part of us that fears primitive threats and responds to them through the emotion of fear. If we allow fear to take over then we will inhibit our recovery since, as you learned, recovery happens in a parasympathetic state of relaxation. Sure, sometimes fear is appropriate as it can encourage us to take action, but allowing fear to dictate our future prevents us from maintaining that natural condition of health.

Performance anxiety and fear can wreak havoc on any performer or athlete that has faced a physical challenge, if it is not addressed competently. I know that it is not always easy to ask for support, especially when it comes to your mental and emotional well-being. Unfortunately, as athletes we are taught to be "tough" in all circumstances. Sometimes being tough can also mean asking for the help you need. That is why I want to extend my time to you outside of this book and offer my support for your journey. If learning the Injured to Elite method has not fully equipped you to overcome this, then send an email to davemeyer@plperform for a free consultation.

Staying On Track

The first section of this book was devoted to the philosophy and mentality it takes to go from injured to elite. The book was not organized this way by mistake — everything has to start with the mind. A conversation I had with John Denney prior to writing this book reminds me of this story: When I was falling a bit off-track with some of my performance-oriented goals, John asked if I was consistent with my meditation. I told him that I was continuing to meditate but the other positive habits I had developed were beginning to lack consistency.

John challenged me, he said: "I bet meditation was the first to go!" His advice was to stay consistent and prioritize my meditation which would allow the rest to fall into place. If you are lacking harmony and peace then there is no better way to attain it again then by being more consistent with your meditation. Is this happening to you? Take action now! Put meditation right at the top of your performance journal priority list; don't wait until tomorrow morning. Make the change immediately. Remember the law of momentum? It starts with the first step. Don't make the excuse that you don't have the time, that just means you're not prioritizing properly. When it feels like you're drowning in commitments, that's when you need the most meditation.

Speaking of recovery, that innate process which occurs in our body with proper sleep and nutrition, allowing for it should be a priority as well. Besides getting adequate sleep and feeding yourself the right type of fuel, it is so important to schedule off-days; real off-days, not a full day of non-sports errands and chores. If you do not have the luxury to give yourself full off-days in-season, then at least take scale-back days when you can take most activities off your plate for the day. But let's really be honest, unless you are in real battle as a soldier or fighting for your life, is there really no way to get a day off? Taking that day off will allow you to have the game or workout of your life next time because it allowed you to fully recharge your batteries and return at full force.

The best way to ensure taking days off is to schedule them ahead of time whenever possible. This is similar to vacation at a day job; many hard-working employees out there don't take their vacations because they think there's some sort of status in working themselves to illness, while others simply don't ask for it ahead of time and can't get the days they want so close to the dates. When you run yourself into the ground and need to ask for a day off without proper notice, you are only setting yourself up for failure. Don't use vacation or off-days and plan to need to use sick days in the near future; it is always better to use vacation days rather than sick days! No one likes to be sick. So keep on top of your recovery and use those scheduled days off, and you'll need less sick days.

CHAPTER 10
CONCLUSION

Congratulations! That is all there is to it. Through the Injured to Elite process, you discovered the silver lining to one of your darkest moments and found empowerment in all aspects of your life. Best of all, no hand holding was really necessary; this book provided some guidance, but you did all the work yourself. And indeed, you were all that you needed.

In this sometimes short-sighted and superficial world, whether you play a professional sport on the big screen, or jog around the block before work in the morning, everyone requires a higher purpose. Competing against others, or even ourselves, is not enough since it rarely contributes to the greater good; winning is just not enough.

The intent of this book is not to put you on a mission to start the next world-changing non-profit (though I'd be glad if you do), rather it is to use a physical challenge as a means to re-focus, and define who you are, above and beyond your injury and physical performance. Though I've mentioned all this before, it's normal if it hasn't sunk in yet. And if you had a realization reading that last section a few seconds ago, wonderful! You might just be starting the journey of finding your higher purpose. As the author of this book, I am truly inspired that you've read it and have gotten a start on making this transformation; you are the hero here, the one I am rooting for!

When we find higher purpose in our struggles, we can then truly make a dent on this universe. Perhaps you started reading this book looking for a roadmap to your own body. To that end, I presented you with our innate ability to tap into a natural power we possess (a gift to you, of yourself). Sure, some science was involved in the performance optimization chapter, but I suspect it wasn't anything all that foreign to you. You see, your clinician or performance experts are no smarter than you. We all just chose different career and life paths.

Still, you've probably not been encouraged to take ownership of your body and mind by the many professionals you sought out. Maybe they wanted to keep the upper-hand because they don't realize that you taking ownership here doesn't mean abandoning them, it means that you do the work to understand the three tenets of evidence-based medicine (the clinician, the research, and your own experience), and take the initiative to lead your recovery and post-injury life. Much of the medical research and knowledge out there is available for the taking, and it doesn't require an M.D. In fact, it should be every medical professional's job to share and interpret that wealth of knowledge and experience for you, the patient. This very book is part of that. It isn't a medical how-to guide, nor the latest trendy self-help tome, nor is it even a workout program. This wasn't about learning how to complete your New Year's resolution of losing the 30 pounds, or how to rehab your knee or shoulder quicker. My mission is to see a dramatic shift in the structure of health care and sports performance where you are the hero, not us.

I know that it would be naïve of me to believe that my words alone will be enough, so I am calling on you, and every other reader to action. Spread the word to others that they are in the driver's seat and can use their own challenges, physical or otherwise, to better everything around them. Spread that same word to your healthcare and performance professionals in this time of change in the healthcare industry. Tell them how much you appreciate their guidance, but also remind them that you are taking the lead here. Inspire us medical professionals to further inspire others by sharing the Injured to Elite method.

Do not let your suffering or fear stand in the way of the life that you have been presented. The gift, which has been given to you after injury, will serve as an infinite source of power to not just overcome physical challenges, but to propel you into a greater and fuller life. Accept this gift and never look back!

I want to thank all of those along my journey that have inspired me to realize the Injured to Elite method. To all of the teachers, professors, loved ones, and colleagues that challenged me throughout my life, thank you. And most of all, thank you to all of my patients and clients over the years. Thank you for letting me challenge you, and for not giving up on yourself. In times of darkness in your life, I feel blessed to have been connected with each and every one of you — I will never stop rooting for you! And most of all, I will never stop being inspired by the sheer willpower that we possess as humans to turn tragedy into triumph.

Thank you to my father, Dean Meyer who taught me to never allow physical circumstances to define a life. His legacy lives on in the Injured to Elite way and this book is dedicated to his 52 years of life on this earth.

And thank you to the New York Mets for giving my father a way to "Always Believe!"

THANK YOU

REFERENCES

Brumitt, J., En Gilpin, H., Brunette, M., & Meira, E. P. (2010). Incorporating kettlebells into a lower extremity sports rehabilitation program. *North American journal of sports physical therapy* : NAJSPT, 5(4), 257–265.

Christopher J. May, Brian D. Ostafin & Evelien Snippe (2020) The relative impact of 15-minutes of meditation compared to a day of vacation in daily life: An exploratory analysis, *The Journal of Positive Psychology*, 15:2, 278-284, DOI: 10.1080/17439760.2019.1610480

Freburger, J. K., Holmes, G. M., Agans, R. P., Jackman, A. M., Darter, J. D., Wallace, A. S., Castel, L. D., Kalsbeek, W. D., & Carey, T. S. (2009). The rising prevalence of chronic low back pain. *Archives of internal medicine*, 169(3), 251–258. https://doi.org/10.1001/archinternmed.2008.543

Goldsby, T. L., Goldsby, M. E., McWalters, M., & Mills, P. J. (2017). Effects of Singing Bowl Sound Meditation on Mood, Tension, and Well-being: An Observational Study. *Journal of Evidence-Based Complementary & Alternative Medicine*, 22(3), 401–406. https://doi.org/10.1177/2156587216668109

Gruzelier, John. (2013). EEG-neurofeedback for optimising performance. I: A review of cognitive and affective outcome in healthy participants. *Neuroscience and biobehavioral reviews*. 44. 10.1016/j.neubiorev.2013.09.015.

Hilton, L., Hempel, S., Ewing, B. A., Apaydin, E., Xenakis, L., Newberry, S., Colaiaco, B., Maher, A. R., Shanman, R. M., Sorbero, M. E., & Maglione, M. A. (2017). Mindfulness Meditation for Chronic Pain: Systematic Review and Meta-analysis. Annals of behavioral medicine : a publication of the *Society of Behavioral*

Medicine, 51(2), 199–213. https://doi.org/10.1007/s12160-016-9844-2

Kaul, P., Passafiume, J., Sargent, C. R., & O'Hara, B. F. (2010). Meditation acutely improves psychomotor vigilance, and may decrease sleep need. *Behavioral and brain functions* : BBF, 6, 47. https://doi.org/10.1186/1744-9081-6-47

Lohr, B. A., & Scogin, F. (1998). Effects of self-administered visuo-motor behavioral rehearsal on sport performance of collegiate athletes. Journal of Sport Behavior, 21(2), 206–218.

Lorenz, Dan & Reiman, Michael (2011) "Integration of Strength and Conditioning Principles into a Rehabilitation Program" *International Journal of Sports Physical Therapy* 6(3): 241-53.

Mazaud-Guittot, S., Kristiansen, K., Brunak, S., Kjaer, M., Juul, A., & Jégou, B. (2018). Ibuprofen alters human testicular physiology to produce a state of compensated hypogonadism. *Proceedings of the National Academy of Sciences of the United States of America*, 115(4), E715–E724. https://doi.org/10.1073/pnas.1715035115

Meigh, N. J., Keogh, J., Schram, B., & Hing, W. A. (2019). Kettlebell training in clinical practice: a scoping review. *BMC sports science, medicine & rehabilitation*, 11, 19. https://doi.org/10.1186/s13102-019-0130-z

Milewski MD, Skaggs DL, Bishop GA, et al. (2014). Chronic lack of sleep is associated with increased sports injuries in adolescent athletes. J Pediatr Orthop. 34(2):129-133. doi:10.1097/BPO.0000000000000151

Piana LE, Garvey KD, Burns H, Matzkin EG. The Cold, Hard Facts of Cryotherapy in Orthopedics. Am J Orthop (Belle Mead NJ). 2018;47(9):10.12788/ajo.2018.0075. doi:10.12788/ajo.2018.0075

Kristensen, D. M., Desdoits-Lethimonier, C., Mackey, A. L., Dalgaard, M. D., De Masi, F., Munkbøl, C. H., Styrishave, B., Antignac, J. P., Le Bizec, B., Platel, C., Hay-Schmidt, A., Jensen, T. K., Lesné, L.,

www.angeladuckworth.com/grit-scale

From Dr. Coppola's 2013 article "Thought Viruses" which can be found here: https://drdavidcoppola.com/wp-content/uploads/2016/08/Thought-Viruses.pdf

More details on thought viruses can be found at the noijam blog: https://noijam.com/2016/03/09/thought-viruses/

The STOP-Bang website was put up by a research team at the University of Toronto: http://www.stopbang.ca/osa/screening.php

ABOUT THE AUTHOR

Dr. David Meyer is a Sports Performance-oriented Physical Therapist that graduated with his Doctorate in Physical Therapy from New York University. After completing an advanced sports residency training program at the world-renowned Hospital for Special Surgery in New York, he served as the Medical and Rehabilitation Coordinator for the St. Louis Cardinals for three years from 2015 through the 2017 season. This was a dream of his that came to fruition 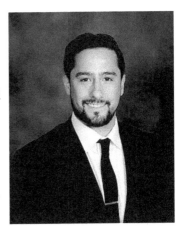 after playing baseball throughout his entire life into the collegiate level. During his time working for the Cardinals he discovered a new appreciation for the psychological implications of sports rehabilitation after seeing the profound impact it had on players, and began developing a comprehensive approach to integrating mental skills and strategies into the physical rehabilitation process.

While now serving as an advocate for athletes going through adversity and working towards advanced credentials with the Association of Applied Sports Psychology, as a Certified Mental Performance Consultant, his mission has become to "Empower those facing physical challenges to transform their lives through an optimal state of body, mind, and spirit." Currently he resides in New York with his soon-to-be wife (wedding was delayed by COVID). David integrates all of the principles he shares in this book into his own physical and mental routine as he continually strives for personal and professional growth. He can be reached on social media @davemmeyer and through e-mail at davemeyer@plperform.com with any inquires.

Made in USA - North Chelmsford, MA
1178378_9780578712000
10.12.2020 0818